"Paramedic Kevin Grange has taken us on an insightful and tumultuous virtual journey that reveals the challenging rites of passage needed to become a paramedic. Come along for the ride, you will be inspired."
—Richard H. Carmona, MD, MPH, FACS,
Seventeenth Surgeon General of the United States

"In his powerful memoir, *Lights and Sirens: The Education of a Paramedic*, Kevin Grange gives the public a raw, yet intimate view of the making of a paramedic on the gritty streets of Los Angeles. Throughout the narrative, Grange beautifully captures the emotions of his successes and failures as he tries to perfect the art of saving lives. His personal story within these pages is riveting and will only add to the legend of the first responder."
—Paul A. Ruggieri, MD, author of
Confessions of a Surgeon and *The Cost of Cutting*

"*Lights and Sirens* is as fast-paced and thrilling as a ride along in a speeding ambulance. Kevin Grange takes you with him as he discovers the challenge, excitement, and stress of training to be a paramedic on the streets of Los Angeles."
—Judy Melinek, MD, *New York Times* bestselling coauthor of
*Working Stiff: Two Years, 262 Bodies and
the Making of a Medical Examiner*

"Kevin Grange's *Lights and Sirens* is an authentic, compelling narrative of Grange's journey through UCLA paramedic school and field internship on Los Angeles's dangerous streets as he trains to save the lives of victims of heart attack, stroke, and trauma. Grange is an excellent writer who does a great service to his new profession in conveying not just the accurate details and heart-pounding excitement of the job, but also revealing the essential compassion of the truest caregivers. *Lights and Sirens* is a book to be appreciated by both the general public and the fire and emergency medical services community."
—Peter Canning, author of *Paramedic: On the Front Lines of Medicine*

Lights

&

Sirens

The Education of a Paramedic

Kevin Grange

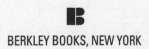

BERKLEY BOOKS, NEW YORK

BERKLEY

An imprint of Penguin Random House LLC
375 Hudson Street, New York, New York 10014

This book is an original publication of Penguin Random House LLC.

Library of Congress Cataloging-in-Publication Data

Grange, Kevin.
Lights and sirens : the education of a paramedic / by Kevin Grange. —First edition.
p.   cm.
ISBN 978-0-425-27523-8 (paperback)
1. Grange, Kevin.   2. Emergency medical technicians—California—Los Angeles—Biography.
3. UCLA–Daniel Freeman Paramedic Program—Students—Biography.   4. Emergency medical
technicians—Education—California—Los Angeles.   5. Emergency medicine—Study and
teaching—California—Los Angeles.   6. Medical emergencies—California—Los Angeles.
7. Ambulance service—California—Los Angeles.   I. Title.
RA645.6.C2G73 2015
616.02'5071092—dc23
[B]
2014045101

PUBLISHING HISTORY
Berkley trade paperback edition / June 2015

PRINTED IN THE UNITED STATES OF AMERICA

10 9 8 7 6 5 4 3 2 1

Cover photos: (front) Mike Powell / Getty Images; (back): welcomia / Shutterstock.
Cover design by Edwin Tse.
Interior text design by Kelly Lipovich.
Photo on page 311 by Nanci Medina

This book describes the real experiences of real people. The author has disguised the identities
of some, and in some instances created composite characters, but none of these changes has
affected the truthfulness and accuracy of his story.

*Penguin Random House is committed to publishing works of quality and integrity.
In that spirit, we are proud to offer this book to our readers;
however, the story, the experiences, and the words
are the author's alone.*

Penguin
Random
House

*This book is dedicated to my loving family,
with infinite gratitude.*

Contents

Three | *Field Internship*

Introduction

The fate of the wounded rests with the one who
applies the first dressing.

—*Nicholas Senn, MD*

The 911 call came in on a Friday night in the summer of 2011 from a gritty part of Los Angeles known on the street as Ghost Town. As usual, it was a trauma. At the fire station on the corner of 124 East I Street and Avalon Boulevard, the lights flickered briefly, followed by the alarm tones, and then moments later, dispatch broadcast over the loudspeaker: *"Engine and rescue. A stabbing."*

In the upstairs bunkroom where he'd been resting, firefighter/paramedic Tim Hill leapt from his bed, sprinted to the fire pole, and began sliding down. The call also roused two other firefighters, who slid down immediately after Tim, and three more from the TV room downstairs, who hustled into the garage bay. And with that, Station 38 of the Los Angeles Fire Department woke to life: the lights on the apparatus floor blinked on, the station doors opened, and six firefighters could be seen stepping into rubber insulated boots, pulling up yellow turnout pants, and throwing on brush coats. The men moved with speed and precision, the result of years on the job.

And then there was me—the paramedic intern.

I'd just finished showering and was standing half-dressed in the upstairs locker room when the tones first went off. Before I even heard the nature of the call, I threw on a shirt, grabbed my watch, and tore down the hall. Forbidden to use the fire pole as an intern, I instead hurtled down the stairs toward the garage bay. A fall down those stairs would break my bones and knock me unconscious—but far worse would be watching the ambulance leave without me. Just the week before, a classmate of mine who'd been interning here on another shift had missed a call—a double shooting at a recreation center—and I hadn't seen him since. No one had said anything but I didn't need to ask. Miss a call during your field internship of paramedic school and you're gone.

In the garage bay, the fire engine pulled out and I picked up the pace, leaping down the last five steps and sprinting across the apparatus floor to the ambulance.

Tim hopped into the driver's seat of the ambulance and hit the ignition. Firefighter/paramedic Eddie Higgins slid into the passenger seat next to Tim, radioed to dispatch that we were en route, and grabbed the map book. Tim shifted into drive, easing his foot off the brake.

I grabbed my gear, jumped into the back of the slow-rolling ambulance, and hollered, "I'm here!" Settling into the captain's seat, I yanked my turnouts on over my shorts and buckled my seat belt. Tim pulled out onto the street and activated the emergency lights—red and white LEDs flashing in 360 degrees. Less than three minutes had elapsed since the tones sounded and an anxious sweat had already replaced the dampness from my shower. The station doors thundered closed behind us and Rescue Ambulance 38 pulled out into the dark streets of L.A.

Tim turned left on I Street, made a right on Avalon Boulevard, and floored it. Eddie activated the siren, its loud wail rising and falling like a sea swell. In the back, I threw on my safety glasses and

EMS exam gloves and scanned the dispatch information on the small computer screen to my right: *18 y/o male. Life status questionable. Location of assailant unknown.* I struggled to slow my breath and recalled the first steps of treating a pulseless stabbing victim in the field: ensure scene safety; start CPR; plug the holes; and, if a heartbeat returned, apply "diesel therapy," aka haul ass to the hospital.

As the ambulance raced toward the intersection of Avalon and the Pacific Coast Highway—a stretch home to liquor stores, weekly motels, and junkyards—Tim blasted the air horn and Eddie cycled the siren, switching its wail to a high-pitched yelp. Some cars pulled right. Some turned left. Some slammed on their brakes and others had absolutely no frickin' idea there was an ambulance driving Code 3 behind them.

"Clear right!" yelled Eddie, scanning the intersection and pointing to a pickup truck to pull over.

Tim weaved through the mess, turned right on the PCH, and hit the gas.

In most places in America, summer means family vacations, lemonade stands, and swimming lessons at the local pool. But not in Ghost Town. Here, summer means the arrival of "shooting season," when tempers rise with the temperature. Gangbangers stay out later. Drink more liquor. Sell more guns, deal more drugs, and create a drastic spike in emergencies between July and September. Tonight's assailant could be someone from the Ghost Town Bloods, Harbor City Crips, or Westside Wilmas. Or it might be someone from the Eastside Wilmas, Ghost Town Locos, or Harbor City Rifas. For years they'd been fighting to control Ghost Town's gun and narcotic trade, occasionally catching kids in their crossfire. Then again, tonight's assailant could also turn out to just be some girl on meth who caught her guy cheating and confronted him in the kitchen.

Tim took a left on a dark residential street and Eddie cut the siren, leaving only our emergency lights splashing red across the rows of single-story homes with barred windows and security doors. At the far end of the street, I saw Engine 38 parked beside a half dozen cop cars, illuminated by the twitchy spotlight of a police helicopter scanning the area.

I said a quick prayer for safety. Slid over to the bench seat near the back door and checked my gear. Tim navigated the ambulance past the police cars and parked in front of the engine. The door locks popped open and I jumped out to a sudden assault of sound—cops talking, radios squawking, a police helicopter, aka "ghetto bird," buzzing overhead, and my captain, Chase Turner, hurrying over with the scene "size-up."

"Sounds like we have two patients and we're going to the second floor of that apartment building," he said, pointing. "PD has cleared us to enter."

The second floor, I thought, cursing my luck. Assault victims never collapsed in well-lit living rooms—they were always in the back bedroom of some upstairs unit with a barking pit bull and no electricity, lying in a red puddle of themselves.

"Let's get moving," I said, pulling out the gurney.

Eddie hustled over. "Tim's got the gurney. Get your gear and hurry up!"

I grabbed the cardiac monitor and first-in bag, which had all the equipment I'd need to save someone's life . . . or determine death. Captain Turner and Eddie led us down a cracked sidewalk that snaked through an overgrown courtyard littered with broken toys and rusted barbecues. Relics of an innocent age. Captain Turner lit the way with a flashlight, and the rest of the firefighters from the engine fell in line behind us.

Eddie hollered to me above the roar of helicopter rotors. "Got your ballistics vest on?"

"I thought it was a stabbing," I said.

"We don't know what we're walking into," he barked. "Haven't you learned by now the only thing dispatch is good for is the address?"

I told Eddie I'd be fine. "PD's cleared us to enter."

Eddie shook his head and pressed on. "Do you feel safe?" he asked.

Is it even possible to feel safe in Ghost Town after dark? I thought. Of course not. But I nodded yes. By the twenty-first shift in my paramedic field internship, not failing took precedence over almost all else.

We arrived at a narrow staircase leading to the second floor and started up. There was the tap-tap sound of tactical boots on metal stairs. A feeling of being watched. Eyes peered out from between window blinds. An eerie calm.

Stillness before the storm.

You got this, I told myself. *Walk in there and get it done.* I'd spent the previous eight grueling months of paramedic school preparing for this moment. I was ready. Yet I also knew I was about to walk into one of the most stressful situations of my life. On a critical trauma call, you have ten minutes to get on and off scene. The goal is to arrive, treat any immediate life threats, then get patients loaded up and en route to the hospital so they can be under the surgeon's knife within the "golden hour." And already the clock was ticking. Already we were behind the eight ball and struggling to catch up.

We reached the top of the stairs and headed for an apartment at the end of a dark hallway. The carpet was stained and smelled of puke and piss. I walked in time with Captain Turner and Eddie. Together, they had more than forty years of experience working for the Los Angeles Fire Department. Ballistics vest or no vest—I'd follow those guys into anything. But, as we arrived at apartment 2D, both stepped aside.

"After you," said Captain Turner, motioning me ahead.

Eddie took the cardiac monitor from me. "Run your call. We're right behind you."

I shuffled past them, knocked twice, and yelled "Paramedics!" The door opened and then it came—chaos. A stereo blasting, the propulsive, flashing images of a fifty-inch TV, and a swarm of teenagers shouting:

"Help them!"

"Do something!"

"Hurry!"

In I went, into the living room, where one teenage boy was reclined on the couch, his face wrinkled in pain, his right hand pressed against his stomach, his legs limp like a puppet with cut strings. I set down my equipment and yelled to Eddie, "Let's clear the room. Turn off the TV. And get some lights on!"

"Done!" Eddie yelled back. "You have a patient in the kitchen, too."

Another boy, about the same age, was half standing in the kitchen. I couldn't see his face. His legs were wobbly and his upper body was slumped over the counter for support. There was blood on the back of his shirt between his shoulder blades. I directed one of the firefighters to assess him. "Let me know what you got."

I set the first-in bag down next to my patient. I knelt down and Tim crouched behind me. He'd brought the gurney to the bottom of the apartment stairs, then hurried up after us. As my two preceptors, Tim and Eddie's job was to watch me run the call. Grade my every move. Analyze each word. And jump in the moment I got off track.

"What's your plan?" Tim asked, leaning in.

"START triage," I said, grabbing my stethoscope.

START, which stands for "simple triage and rapid treatment" is a way of quickly and effectively determining the severity of patients' injuries in a multiple casualty incident, or anytime the number of patients might exceed the medical resources on scene. When you're responsible for triage and your motor's revved, START teaches, remember RPM. Respirations. Perfusion. Mental status. Is the patient breathing more than thirty times per minute? Is perfusion, or blood flow, compromised—as evidenced by no pulse at the wrist? Does the patient's mental status allow him or her to follow simple commands? If there is a deficit in any of these, the patient is critical—a "red tag" who needs immediate lifesaving interventions and transport.

"Good," said Tim. "Get it done!"

By now, Captain Turner and the guys on the engine had cleared the room and the lights were on. The apartment was full of empty beer cans, playing cards, and ashtrays. The gray carpet was sprinkled with blood. I knelt down and introduced myself to the boy on the couch. "What's your name?" I asked.

"Javier," he said, wincing in pain and offering me his hand.

"While I check your pulse, can you tell me what year it is?"

"Two thousand eleven."

I relayed my findings to Tim. "His airway's clear, but his breathing is shallow and rapid." I asked a firefighter to my left to put Javier on oxygen via a non-rebreather mask at 15 liters per minute and continued my assessment. I checked Javier's radial pulse on his wrist—strong and rapid. His skin was pink, warm, and sweaty. Was his heart rate elevated from the pain? Or was it trying to compensate for internal blood loss?

Javier lifted his shirt. "He stabbed me, man. He *stabbed* me!"

I saw a single puncture wound with a slab of fatty tissue protruding on the lower right quadrant, near the appendix, small intestine, and ascending colon. I was relieved to see the bleeding was controlled but, still, it didn't look good.

"Were you stabbed anywhere else?"

"No, man," Javier uttered. "We were just havin' a party and he got all crazy."

"What do you want to do?" said Tim, interjecting. "You have two patients. Speed it up. Make decisions."

I told Tim there was no deficit to RPM, but I was calling Javier a red tag. "I'm worried about internal injuries. He's got a rapid pulse so I'm afraid he's compensating and could deteriorate."

"Or he might just be in pain," replied Tim. "But better to over-triage. How long was the knife?" he asked the patient.

Javier motioned with his hands—about the size of a Buck knife. "But I don't think it went all the way in."

I turned to one of the firefighters and asked him to get me a set of vital signs.

Suddenly Eddie yelled from across the room: "I have a critical patient here. I need a set of ears!"

I grabbed my stethoscope and hurried over. Eddie and Bryan, a firefighter off the engine, were kneeling next to the other boy, who now sat on a kitchen chair. His skin was pale, cool, and moist. Eddie had cut off his shirt and placed him on oxygen. Two stab wounds decorated his back: one below his right shoulder blade and a second wound a few inches below that, where Bryan was now applying a gauze dressing.

I handed Eddie my stethoscope and he quickly inserted the earbuds and placed the bell of the stethoscope on the boy's chest to assess breathing. The boy breathed in and out a few times, as if gathering up energy to speak. "My . . . name . . . is . . . Oscar . . ." he whispered, speaking in short, clipped, one-word bursts.

Forget perfusion and mental status, I thought, *Eddie's right, this guy's critical!*

"I've got diminished lung sounds on the right," Eddie said, yanking off the stethoscope. "Could be a pneumothorax."

"Let's call for a second ambulance and get the stair chair," I announced.

"Already done!" replied Eddie. "This guy's mine. I called for medical aid the moment we walked in the door," he told me.

Just then, another firefighter appeared with the stair chair—a collapsible aluminum seat that allows EMS to move patients down stairs without lifting them. Bryan and I carried Oscar to the chair, fastened two seat belts across his chest, and wheeled him to the door.

Down below, two paramedics from Station 85 in nearby Harbor City appeared with their gurney.

Bryan went out into the hallway to assist with the foot section of the chair. I took the handlebars near Oscar's head and tilted the stair chair back to lift the front wheels and clear the doorway.

"I'll handle that," Eddie said to me, hustling over. "Get back to your patient."

As he said this, the scene screeched to a halt. Had I made a mistake?

I shook it off and raced over to Javier, whose condition was improving. His skin color was better with the oxygen, and the vital signs the firefighter relayed to me were within normal limits. The plan: move him to the stair chair, get him into the back of the ambulance, and do all other treatments en route.

Tim agreed. "Which hospital?"

"A penetrating injury to the torso is trauma center criteria," I said, doing a rapid physical exam of Javier to make sure I hadn't missed anything. "Our closest is Harbor-UCLA."

"Good."

When a firefighter returned with the stair chair, we moved Javier down the stairs and onto the gurney. Up ahead, Rescue Ambulance 85 activated its emergency lights and pulled out with Oscar in the back. Eddie sat in the driver's seat of our ambulance, Rescue 38, with the engine on. Tim and I loaded Javier in the back and closed the doors. "Harbor-UCLA. Code 3," I announced.

Eddie nodded. Hit the lights. Shifted into drive and off we raced.

We had a short ETA to the hospital so I had to work fast. I switched Javier's oxygen line from the tank on the stretcher to the one on the ambulance; started an IV; disposed of the needle in the sharps container; hung an IV bag of normal saline; and placed a pulse oximeter on his finger to measure the amount of oxygen in his blood. It was hard keeping my balance as the ambulance slammed over potholes and veered around impossible corners— gotta love gurney surfing at seventy mph.

Next, I gathered information about Javier's medical history, allergies, and medications; called the ER with my radio report; obtained another set of vitals; listened to lung sounds again; and reassessed his injury as we pulled into the ambulance bay at the hospital. The final push now: I quickly switched his oxygen back to the gurney, tucked in the blood pressure and pulse oximetry cables so they didn't get caught in the gurney wheels, and threw my trash in the tiny receptacle next to the bench seat. Eddie opened the back doors and a rush of warm night air filled the patient compartment.

"Still okay, Javier?" I asked as we pulled him out.

Thumbs-up and a nod.

Harbor-UCLA Medical Center is a 553-bed, acute care facility on the corner of West Carson Street and South Vermont in Torrance. It is the only Level 1 trauma center in the South Bay and Greater Long Beach area and its patient population is as diverse and anxious and impatient as the lunchtime crowd at the Department of Motor Vehicles . . . give or take a stabbing or a gunshot wound or two.

We wheeled Javier through the ambulance bay, teeming with units arriving and departing, and then through the hospital doors, where a heavyset security guard rose from her seat and said to me, "Not so fast, young man. I gotta scan him for weapons first." The security guard passed the wand over the contours of Javier's body before clearing us to enter. "Follow the red line of paint on the floor to the ER."

Tim and I pushed the gurney, following Eddie down long, maze-like hallways. Moments later, we entered through two large white doors and into the bright, busy ER. A triage nurse directed us to an open bed where a trauma team of doctors and nurses waited.

"Tell me when to start talking," I announced loudly, as Tim and I transferred Javier to the bed using the sheet below him.

"Go!" said the doctor.

"We have an eighteen-year-old male, chief complaint right lower quadrant pain, secondary to being stabbed," I began. "Patient states the knife was approximately four inches long but he doesn't think it went in all the way. Upon our arrival, patient was seated on a couch in moderate distress . . ."

And so it went.

The moment I finished, nurses and ER technicians rushed in to remove Javier's clothes, patch him up on the cardiac monitor, obtain vitals and lab samples, and start another IV. The doctor thanked us. "We'll take it from here." We stepped back and a curtain whisked closed in front of us. The call was over.

Sort of.

During field internship, the call still had to be documented on paramedic school paperwork, discussed, analyzed, and assessed with my preceptors. These discussions had the power to fill me with sheer exuberance—or deep depression. Over my first twenty shifts, I realized Tim and Eddie's assessment of my performance on a call could roughly be determined by where I found them immediately after a run. Were they chatting amiably with other EMTs and paramedics in the ambulance bay? A good sign. Were they sitting in the front cab, texting their wives a quick good night? Even better. And if they were using their phones to look up the nearest frozen yogurt shop to stop at on the way home, I'd totally rocked it.

That night, Tim and Eddie waited for me behind the ambulance with their arms folded across their chests. It was as if they were trying to get as far as possible from the radio in the front cab, lest it accidentally record the reprimand that was to occur.

"How'd you think the call went?" Tim asked as I arrived.

First I listed the good points: I'd created a workable scene for myself, assessed and treated Javier correctly—even nailing the IV on an especially bouncy section of road—I'd chosen the right hospital, and I gave solid reports to both the nurse over the radio and to the doctors at the hospital.

Eddie cut me off. "But you missed the critical patient on scene!"

"I thought if I delegated assessing the second patient to a firefighter, we could work faster," I replied.

Eddie said that, as lead paramedic on the call, I must take responsibility for both patients initially. "You should've done a quick RPM check on both patients, stayed with the one that was more critical, and then delegated the other patient to us."

I asked Eddie when he'd thought to call for a second ambulance and get the stair chair.

"The moment I walked in the door," he replied, noting the importance of taking visual vital signs. "I saw that kid's bad skin signs and work of breathing from across the room and called immediately."

Eddie stormed off, his face red with anger. He always got mad when a call wasn't run perfectly, but I appreciated the standards he held me to, and that he maintained himself. Tim and I finished cleaning the gurney, applied a fresh set of sheets, and loaded it back into the ambulance. "Keep your head up," he said. "You're putting the pieces together, moving faster and making solid treatment decisions."

I thanked Tim for his encouragement and Eddie, too, when I hopped back into the rig. We cleared from the hospital fifteen minutes after we'd moved Javier to an ER bed and transferred care to the hospital. It was early Saturday morning now. As we drove south on the 110 Freeway back to the neighborhood of Wilmington, I leaned back in the captain's seat, flicked off the lights in the patient compartment, and relished the air-conditioned darkness and the vastness of Los Angeles reduced to the two small ambulance windows. At night, the lights muted and merged and the city seemed to float in the L.A. basin like a magic carpet of color. Gazing out, it was hard to believe there were people out there suffering. Hurting each other. Heroin running into veins. Guns popping. Cars colliding. And hearts stopping. I closed my eyes—exhausted after twenty hours on the job—and let the stressful sights and sounds from the stabbing call run off me like wastewater.

I was half-asleep when Tim exited off the 110 and turned left on the PCH. It was about that time that a forty-year-old man on North Lagoon Avenue suddenly woke up with a sharp burning sensation in his chest, like someone was stabbing a cigarette into his left coronary artery. His wife turned on the light next to the bed, grabbed the phone, and dialed three digits.

We were five blocks from the station when I felt the ambulance suddenly accelerate. I blinked my eyes open: red emergency lights, followed by our sirens, the air horn, and a sharp U-turn.

"Hang on," yelled Tim. "We just got another call."

Every year in the United States, hundreds of emergency medical technicians (EMTs) enroll in paramedic school with hopes of earning their paramedic licenses and becoming certified as one of the most advanced emergency medical services providers. Often used interchangeably with the term "prehospital care," EMS covers the assessment and treatment of ill or injured patients in an out-of-hospital setting (typically while also en route to an appropriate medical facility), and paramedics are at the front of the lines.

I hadn't followed a traditional route to paramedic school. After graduating with a creative writing degree from Seattle University, I initially worked in business development for a real estate company in Orange County, California, and spent my free time writing and pursuing my love of the outdoors. I enjoyed my life. The money was decent. I traveled around the world, published a few freelance articles, and even wrote a book about a twenty-four-day "Snowman Trek" through the Himalayan kingdom of Bhutan that received a half-page review in the *Wall Street Journal*. But I longed to help people in a more direct and meaningful way.

It was 2007 when I first thought of becoming a paramedic, but my fascination with emergency medicine had begun many years earlier. I remember being around four years old and kicking my legs with excitement in the car when I heard sirens or when my parents said, "Look, a fire truck!" In the years that followed, toy fire engines responded to the mass casualty incidents I staged in my living room, and there was nothing better than visiting the local fire station, sitting on the ladder truck, and having the captain give me a sticker badge. While the sticker badges faded from my T-shirts with repeated washings in the laundry, my interest in the fire department endured. It deepened when I was in third grade and my family moved to New Hampshire, where we lived with my grandparents for a year. Their house sat directly across the street from the Newfields Fire Station, a white, barnlike structure that housed a single fire engine. The Newfields Fire Department was staffed by volunteers who were notified of a call by an alarm that sat atop a telephone pole in front of the station. When a call came in, the alarm broadcast its wake-up-the-dead wail clear across town and rattled the windows of my grandparents' house.

For most people in Newfields, a small town along the Squamscott River, that fire alarm was dreadful. When it rang, drivers rolled up their car windows and sped out of sight. Children fled the nearby playground, as if the sound was a swarm of bees, and I'm sure many living room rugs discovered how scared the family dog was. But for me, that alarm was like hearing my favorite song come on over the radio. The moment it sounded, I'd hurry to the wooden fence that enclosed my grandparents' yard and watch the firefighters arrive at the station. Within moments, they'd race up in pickup trucks (usually with an emergency light on the dash), trailing great clouds of dust. With the greatest longing, I'd watch them dress in their turn-outs, climb aboard the engine, and then zoom off. What adventures awaited those men and women! What danger! What glory! And what companionship held them together, like soldiers. To this day, the sight of a fire truck responding to a call has never filled me with sadness or annoyance or made me think, "Someone must be having a really bad day"—I've always thought instead, "someone must have great hope because help is on the way." While the first word of an incident might be tragic or traumatic—be it a heart attack or a mass shooting—the final statement will always be one of heroic emergency response. The police, a fire engine, and an ambulance will respond. The American flag will shine amid the smoke, and the boots on the ground will belong to brave men and women who have arrived to help.

Those childhood memories came back to me one night in 2007 as I lay on a bed in a San Diego emergency room. Earlier that evening, I'd been to a concert and had passed out in the parking lot from dehydration. My friend called 911 and, moments later, an engine and ambulance roared up. I remember three distinct things from that evening: First, the strange sensation of suddenly finding myself on the ground with no idea how I'd gotten there. Second, how comforting it felt to see a paramedic and his team of firefighters helping me as I slowly came around, and letting me know they'd be taking good care of me. And third, as we drove to the hospital (and I began feeling better), being thoroughly impressed with the paramedic's professionalism. As he relayed his findings to our destination hospital and treated the dehydration that had caused my fainting spell, I realized how, within minutes, he and his team had taken my vital signs, ruled out any trauma, placed me on oxygen and a cardiac monitor, checked my blood glucose, given me a neurological function exam, started an IV, given me fluid, and done a 12-lead ECG. In the process, they had ruled out a heart attack, shock, a diabetic emergency, overdose, stroke, cervical spine injury, and seizure. I was amazed at how different the paramedic's speedy treatment was from my primary care physician, who took an hour just to diagnose and treat a sinus infection.

This first encounter with a paramedic as a patient instilled in me a new respect, but I also had to admit I knew nothing about what being a paramedic actually meant. Sure, I knew paramedics saved lives. But how? Did paramedics go to medical school? What was a "typical day at the office" for a paramedic? Did such a thing even exist? Did seeing all that trauma affect their view of the world?

As I left the ER later that night, I resolved to find out more. When I saw the way the paramedics and firefighters worked together as a team and felt the comfort they brought me that night, I grew excited by the possibility of providing that same level of care for others and saving lives. Despite my interest in the fire department as a boy, I'd never really thought seriously about pursuing the profession. It just wasn't something anyone in my family had done before. Maybe it was time I tried something new.

I began my quest by enrolling in a two-day wilderness first aid class, offered by the National Outdoor Leadership School. I figured it would be a good place to start since I spend much of my time outdoors—backpacking, skiing, surfing, and mountain biking. The course gave me an introduction to basic first aid, the initial steps in assessing and treating patients in a wilderness setting, and performing CPR. By the end of the second day, I'd made a host of new friends and received a wilderness-oriented first aid provider card for my wallet. The experience gave me a new bounce to my step and made me want to shout, "I can save a life!"

My obsession with the emergency medical services grew in the months that followed. I read dozens of books and articles about emergency medicine. I enrolled in an emergency medical technician program in Park City, Utah, a 120-hour course consisting of lectures, skills tests, and practical exams. EMT certification is the bare minimum for someone operating an ambulance, and the course taught me basic patient assessment, along with noninvasive skills that focused on the immediate care of critical patients. Following class, I discovered the hardest part about EMS might not be the calls, but rather finding a job. Due to the recession, none of the fire departments or private ambulance companies around Park City were hiring, so I ended up taking a job as a summer EMT at Park City Mountain Resort. There, I responded to mountain biking accidents, hiking incidents, and a few search-and-rescue operations. I also worked as medical assistant at a local family practice, where I gained experience in the clinical setting. When I wasn't working, I pored over EMS books and did a few ride-alongs with the Park City Fire Department.

As I worked in both the field and clinical settings, my passion for "prehospital care" grew and I discovered this branch of medicine was practiced quite differently at various provider levels. Both EMTs and paramedics are trained to respond quickly to medical and traumatic injuries—an EMT operates under a limited scope of practice, whereas a paramedic can deliver more advanced treatments. The scope of practice varies from state to state but, generally speaking, an EMT can assist with a half dozen medications, whereas paramedics have access to more than three times as many possible drugs for their patients. In many places, EMTs can't "break the skin" of a patient, but paramedics can start IVs, give medications via intramuscular injections, test blood sugar, or insert an angiocatheter through the chest wall to reduce the tension built up from a collapsed lung. Paramedics can also do advanced airway maneuvers like inserting a breathing tube down a patient's throat or making a surgical incision under the Adam's apple if needed.

I also found out EMS was delivered to people quite differently, depending on the area and which agency had jurisdiction over the 911 calls. In some places, the fire department responds to all emergencies with an ambulance and fire engine. The ambulance is staffed with either two paramedics, or a paramedic and an EMT. The engine also responds with three or four firefighters, who, depending on the call, also assist with the often overlooked—but ever important—tasks of documentation, interviewing bystanders about the call, crowd control, extricating patients from vehicles, lifting obese patients, or doing chest compressions. In other areas, the fire department doesn't have ambulances as part of its fleet, so private, for-profit ambulance services assist with patient care and transport. Since 80 percent of a fire department's call volume is medical illness or traumatic injury, most firefighters these days have the dual responsibilities of fighting fire and working as EMTs or paramedics.

Despite the complexity on scope of practice, EMS still seemed like the perfect career to me. I enjoy meeting people, hearing their stories, and helping them in a time of need. I also find the human body and medicine immensely interesting. And few jobs in the health care industry are as dynamic as prehospital care. I also loved the team aspect of EMS—working with a crew, the ER staff, and doctors, all toward the common goal of good patient care. And, last, there was just something about holding a radio and saying, "Copy that!" that made me supremely happy. Maybe the radio brought back the innocent walkie-talkie days of my youth. Maybe it meant I was finally realizing my boyhood dream of hopping aboard a fire engine. Or maybe it just symbolized what I've come to hold most sacred in life—people helping people. I had learned a lot about EMS in the two years since that fateful night in the ER in 2007, but I was hungry for more. This left me with one option that filled me with both wild excitement and trepidation—paramedic school.

The jump from being an EMT to a paramedic is the equivalent of transitioning from high school baseball to playing in the majors. While basic treatments must always precede advanced life support interventions and a great EMT can, at times, be more effective than a poor paramedic, the paramedic's scope of practice is simply way beyond an EMTs. A paramedic is the senior medical authority on every emergency scene and has the ultimate decision on patient assessment, treatment, transportation, and hospital destination. Paramedics also make the initial determination about whether to "work up" a cardiac arrest patient on scene, or determine the patient deceased in the field.

In fact, paramedics are held in such high regard by many emergency departments across the country that many doctors now instruct paramedics not to transport a patient in cardiac arrest to the hospital unless they get a pulse back—the message being that if a paramedic can't kick-start a patient's heart in the field, then an emergency room physician won't be able to do it, either.

Every paramedic starts off with at least six months of field experience as an EMT and a valid American Heart Association CPR card. Also required is a driver's license; a high school diploma (at least); and passing a medical physical, an oral interview, and a written entrance exam to paramedic school, a 1,230-plus-hour intense blend of boot camp and medical school. Completion of college-level English, math, anatomy, and physiology courses certainly help, as do classes in medical terminology, ECG (electrocardiogram) interpretation, and pharmacology. And while not an official prerequisite, it's also probably best for everyone if you don't get too freaked out by the sight of severed limbs, protruding bones, bullet holes, blood, vomit, feces, urine, scabies, lice, or bed bugs—

and if you can keep it together when a patient stares you in the eye and says, "Please don't let me die." Over the course of a paramedic's career, he or she will at various points contend with grueling twenty-four-hour shifts, being rookies at a fire station, and learning new treatment protocols and medications, as well as responding to all the urgent calls. And yet none of these experiences matches the stress of paramedic school, where a student must endure all these elements at once—often for the first time—and for months on end.

Paramedic school is divided into three distinct segments. The first part begins with 540 hours of instruction on anatomy and physiology, pathophysiology (the study of disease), and pharmacology, as well as high-stress practical skills tests and emergency scenarios. Next, paramedic students work with patients during grueling tours of duty in local hospitals and trauma centers. During clinical rotations, paramedic students start IVs, give injections, practice intubation, assist with birth, and get a unique, behind-the-scenes look at some of the nation's busiest emergency rooms, labor and delivery wards, operating rooms, and intensive care units. The hours are long and the pace relentless, but both the classroom and the clinical rotations pale in comparison to the last and most difficult part of paramedic school—the field internship. During the field internship, paramedic students work twenty to thirty twenty-four-hour shifts with a local fire department or private ambulance service and struggle to make the difficult and—often traumatizing—transition from the classroom to being street-smart medics. The field internship is where paramedic students discover that while treatment protocols are written in black and white, the job is often a hazy shade of gray. During internship, you not only have to contend with long shifts and being an outsider at a fire station, but also running calls while being graded by two paramedic preceptors. When I asked one graduate what field internship was like, he replied, "Just get kicked in the nuts; it feels about the same."

I heard a lot of horror stories about paramedic school—about panic poops before written tests, sleepless nights on the eve of skills exams, long hours of clinical rotations, and post-traumatic bouts of crying during field internship. And of course, there were countless stories of students failing out. Paramedic school was notorious for straining relationships, or ending them all together. Several people told me paramedic school felt like a college finals week that lasted for nine straight months. Others when asked gave me only a sorry slap on the back and a smile that seemed to say, "You'll see . . ."

Despite these warnings, I was still intent on going to paramedic school. While most graduates said they'd never want to endure it twice, they were also quick to admit the experience was one of the best times of their lives. As I began my research, I looked for a paramedic school with a national reputation. That way, if I applied for jobs out of my region after graduation, my school would have name recognition with employers. I also wanted an institution with a renowned faculty who had time-in-the-trenches experience as paramedics and a school whose graduates had a high success rate on the National Registry Paramedic Exam and were hired quickly after graduation. Lastly, I wanted a paramedic school where my field internship took place in a high-call, urban environment. I wasn't seeking out stabbings, shootings, suicides, car accidents, or the like from a sensationalist point of view—my goal, like a pilot who practices landing his plane in all conditions, was to learn how to run every type of call so that I could become the best paramedic possible.

I discovered many good programs across the country, but the UCLA Paramedic Education Program was my top choice. Originally called the Daniel Freeman Paramedic Program (and still widely known by the name), it was one of the first three paramedic programs in the country, along with one run jointly by the Miami Fire Department and the University of Miami, and Seattle's renowned Medic One program. It was the first in the nation to be nationally accredited and has maintained both a national and international reputation for producing an elite group of professional, critical-thinking medics over the past forty years. Historically, 90 percent of UCLA's paramedic students passed the National Registry qualifying exam the first time and 95 percent were hired within six months of graduation.

I liked, too, that UCLA's Paramedic Education Program didn't exist in isolation, but was part of UCLA's Center for Prehospital Care—a division of the David Geffen School of Medicine that specialized in EMS education, research, and taught over twelve thousand students a year, including members of the FBI, DEA, State Department, U.S. Air Force, U.S. Coast Guard, and fire department personnel from across L.A. County, LAFD, Pasadena, Burbank, Long Beach, Ventura, Santa Monica, Manhattan Beach, and Compton, among others.

I was also impressed that all of the faculty and skills instructors at UCLA were themselves paramedics with years of experience, and that they went above and beyond the national curriculum by certifying students in pediatric advanced life support (PALS), advanced cardiac life support (ACLS), and prehospital trauma life support (PHTLS).

With nearly ten million people—representing 140 different nationalities and speaking 224 different languages—all squeezed into 4,752 square miles, I figured even the slowest day in L.A. was busier than the busiest in many parts of the country. The Los Angeles Fire Department ran over 830 medical and trauma calls a day, virtually ensuring that I'd respond to almost every kind of call. And as an added bonus, if I attended UCLA, I'd be near my family, who had relocated to southern California.

I submitted my application with two letters of recommendation in the spring of 2010 and visited the school in June to take the EMT qualifying exam. Everything about the school felt right—the building and its location, as well as the faculty and prospective students I met. Graduation pictures from almost a half century of classes lined the main hallway and, the moment I saw them, I felt a kind of ownership and pride, and I decided I'd do whatever it took to get my picture on that wall. With that thought driving me, I aced my exam and interview and, by January 2011, found myself headed south on the 405 Freeway early one morning to take my spot in Class 36.

The first part of the drive went smoothly but, as I crossed into the city limits of L.A., my enthusiasm halted with the traffic. Smog blotted out the sun and covered the horizon in an eerie, orange glow. Blown tires and trash littered the highway, and gang graffiti tagged the street signs. Los Angeles no longer felt like the fabled City of Angels, but more like what rapper Dr. Dre declared the "home of drive-bys and AK-matics, swap meets, sticky green and bad traffic" all hovering on the brink of chaos—a gigantic game of Jenga, built by the teetering blocks of race, socioeconomic status, and gang affiliation. Having grown up in a small town in New Hampshire, a place where you didn't lock your front door, I was about to experience a whole new side of life.

As I exited onto Manchester Avenue, heading east toward the paramedic campus in Inglewood, the responsibility suddenly seemed overwhelming and I felt short of breath. In just a few short months, someone in an emergency would call 911 and the fire station I was interning with would respond. No one would arrive before us. No one would arrive with us. Or after us. We would be it. There were no other paramedics warming up like relief pitchers in an EMS bullpen somewhere in case we had a bad day. If we couldn't save the patient's life, it wouldn't be saved, and someone would lose a spouse, a mother, a father, a sibling, a friend . . . or a child.

I tried to psych myself up, as you might in the locker room

before a big game. My brain began a quick list of bullet points to calm my nerves and assure me of success: Captain of high school basketball team? *Check*. Dean's List in college? *Check*. Success in the high-stakes real estate world? *Check*. Guided a twenty-four-day, 216-mile trek through the Himalayas on two separate occasions? *Check*. Published a book? *Check*. And I'd spent nearly every waking moment of the last few years pursuing emergency medicine. Big, bold, underlined *check*.

By the time I pulled into the lot outside the paramedic school, my worries had disappeared. I told myself I would finish paramedic school. And I would not only pass, but I would prevail. I would graduate at the top of my class and be elected valedictorian. I had the maturity. I had the education and I had the experience. Above all, I had the will.

I had no idea.

One | *Classroom*

Next to creating a life, the finest thing a man can do is save one.

—Abraham Lincoln

To know even one life has breathed easier because you have lived—this is to have succeeded.

—Ralph W. Emerson

January

Day One

The UCLA Paramedic Education Program is located on the grounds of the Daniel Freeman Hospital in Inglewood, eleven miles south of UCLA's main campus in the Westwood neighborhood. The Daniel Freeman Hospital itself was closed in 2007 and now serves as a location for television shows and movies shooting medical scenes. The paramedic school occupies the Walter S. Graf Center, a large single-story building on a quiet street of residential homes and a private high school, nestled between the hospital and a helicopter pad—a veritable embodiment of how the profession isn't solely focused on patient care or transportation, but inhabits the dynamic space in between.

I pulled into the parking lot on my first day, already crowded with cars and pickup trucks, many bearing red fire helmet stickers in their back windows. I also noticed two dented vehicles with cracked windshields, which appeared to be abandoned. One car was an old white Toyota. The other was a black Chevrolet *Mo te Car o*, missing letters. I wondered if they'd been left behind by former students who'd crashed and burned out of paramedic school; or maybe they'd been donated by California Highway Patrol for use in extrication scenarios. Either way, I didn't park close, opting for an open space on the other side of the lot. I grabbed my backpack and followed a procession of students V-lining to the door as if it the building was a city bus about to leave without us.

Despite what I'd considered my early arrival, the main classroom was jammed. Two columns of long gray tables stretched from the front of the large classroom to the back. Students sat in blue chairs in pairs of two or three at each table. A large dry erase board hung on the front wall, across which "Welcome, Class 36" had been written in black marker. There was also a podium with a desktop computer and a skeleton model standing in the corner. The skeleton seemed to have a mocking grin, as if he knew something we new students didn't.

I found a seat in back and took stock of my forty other classmates. Almost all guys, except one woman with shoulder-length brown hair who was seated up front. At thirty-six years old, I figured myself likely the oldest student here, by a pretty wide margin. The youngest student I pegged as the kid sitting across from me on the left side of the classroom. With hints of acne dotting his face, he looked as if he'd just traded in his tuxedo from high school prom and caught the first bus to paramedic school. In addition to the woman and the kid, there were eight guys who had clearly been sponsored by their respective fire departments. They all wore black boots, navy blue station uniforms, and shiny badges. The sponsored firefighters would have paramedic school paid for by their departments while earning their regular salaries. Not a bad gig. The rest of us private students wore various manifestations of the school dress code of long pants, close-toed shoes, and collared shirts. And I noticed that everyone was sitting in exactly the same position—with both feet planted firmly on the ground. Spines straight. Hands folded in our laps and a notebook and pen at ready on the desk. It felt like West Point. I half expected a drill sergeant to storm in the room and yell, "Hey, plebe, what's the adult dose of epinephrine in a cardiac arrest? . . . Wrong! . . . A hundred push-ups now!"

At eight a.m., the side door at the front of the classroom opened and Heather Davis appeared. Ms. Davis—as we were to refer to her—was program director for the paramedic school.

"Good morning and welcome to paramedic school," she said with a beaming smile. "I hope you are all as excited as we are to get started."

A registered paramedic with a master's degree in science, Ms. Davis worked in EMS for nearly twenty years in such areas as disaster response, critical incident management, and tactical EMS. Prior to UCLA, she served as education program director for the Los Angeles County Fire Department, where she handled the primary EMT and continuing education programs for over three thousand EMTs and paramedics. She'd been widely published, was a frequent speaker at EMS conferences around the nation, and had recently been named California's EMS Educator of the Year in 2010.

Ms. Davis began with a brief introduction about the philosophy and mission of the program. "We want to carry forward the mission of Daniel Freeman Hospital by providing quality health care with compassion that is inspired by ethical, moral, and human concern for the dignity for each person," she said. "And we want to make a local, national, and international contribution to the field of emergency medicine." From there, Ms. Davis spoke about all the good we'd do as paramedics, helping people in their time of need and saving lives. It was really inspiring stuff, and brought to mind what another paramedic who'd spoken at our earlier orientation had said: "Your patients will be hovering between life and death, and you are going to be the angels that stand in the gap between."

Next, we went around the room and introduced ourselves. Five of the sponsored firefighters were from Los Angeles County Fire Department, three from Santa Monica Fire Department, plus another firefighter from Corona Fire Department, who was paying his own way. The ratio of sponsored firefighters to private students at UCLA varied with every class. In some classes, there were less than five private spots available. Other times—such as our Class 36—private students made up the majority. All of us, of course, had EMT experience (a prerequisite), but even outside of EMS, the students in Class 36 boasted an impressive mix of accomplishments: Among us were ex-Marines, musicians, two former Division 1 soccer players, and a former professional water polo player who'd nearly qualified for the Olympics. One guy, named Patel, had graduated from baking school prior to becoming an EMT, and I learned the young kid sitting across from me was nineteen and named O'Brien. He'd be giving morphine to patients before he could legally drink.

"It's great having you all here," Ms. Davis continued, "and I hope you're ready for an incredible journey."

She handed out our syllabus for the next four months. The syllabus was eleven by seventeen inches, more akin to poster size than a piece of paper, with double-sided printing. The sheer amount of material was jaw-dropping, like four years of med school squeezed into four months.

As Ms. Davis reviewed the course schedule and syllabus, I quickly realized that class in paramedic school was not going to resemble the laid-back lifestyle I'd enjoyed in college. We'd have class from eight a.m. to five p.m. Monday, Tuesday, Thursday, and Friday. There were no lectures scheduled on Wednesdays, but the school would be open for optional study sessions and skills practice. It was clear by the way Ms. Davis said the word "optional," however, that our only option would be to attend.

We'd spend January learning anatomy and physiology (A & P)

and patient assessment. We'd study topical anatomy, the organ systems, bones, major vessels of the body, and, most important, how these systems worked together . . . or didn't.

After A & P, we'd plunge into the "Airway Academy," where we'd learn how to manage a patient's airway and breathing with skills such as endotracheal and nasal intubation (inserting a breathing tube into a patient's windpipe via their mouth or nose) and performing a needle decompression (piercing the chest wall with a needle to relieve the tension built up by a collapsed lung). Following this, medical math would challenge us with long equations, and we'd have exams covering pharmacology, trauma, cardiology, medical emergencies, obstetric emergencies, geriatric patient care, and pediatric patient care.

Over the next four months, we'd endure daily quizzes, lengthy reading assignments each night, online assignments, and monster block exams that detonated like bombs every few weeks. We'd also run emergency scenarios and high-stress skills tests, which one former graduate described as "the only thing that can reduce a grown man to a puddle of nausea, vomiting, and diarrhea."

"Which leads me to my next point," Ms. Davis continued. "How you can be terminated from the program."

The room fell silent.

There were no "gentleman's Cs" in paramedic school. Eighty percent was the minimum passing grade for any quiz, block exam, or skills test. "A student will be terminated if they fail eight quizzes, two block exams, or don't pass the final exam on their first attempt," Ms. Davis explained. Failing any skill three times, or seven individual skills one time, would also get you thrown out. And then, of course, there was the field internship where the ways to get kicked out were simply too numerous to count. For the sponsored guys, failing out would mean returning to their departments, still with a job albeit with their tails between their legs. For the rest of us, failing out meant not only losing both the money we'd spent on tuition and living expenses but also our future careers.

On the encouraging side, Ms. Davis said the UCLA staff would do their best to help us, and added, "We promise to match your energy with our energy." But right then, my "energy" was anxious and worried. My heart raced, and my skin was pale and cool—symptoms of shock.

Ms. Davis seemed to sense a similarly panicked feeling running through the whole class. "Let's take a break," she said, gazing down at her watch. "We'll meet back here in ten minutes."

As students filed out into the hallway, the student sitting next to me leaned over. "What do you call a doctor who graduates from med school with a C average?" he asked.

I shrugged my shoulders.

"You call him doctor," he said. "Not so in paramedic school." He extended his hand. "I'm Wilson."

"Grange," I replied.

Wilson was a blond surfer in his midtwenties who had graduated from University of California at Santa Cruz and spent the last few years working as a lifeguard in Orange County. I liked Wilson immediately but, at the moment, I needed something far more important than friendship—books.

During the break, a line formed outside the large closet that served as the school's bookstore. The shelves were crowded with textbooks for EMT classes, EMT refresher, paramedic preparatory classes, paramedic refresher, pharmacology, and electrocardiography (ECG) interpretation.

"What do you need?" asked Michael Gudger, the school registration coordinator, as I arrived at the front of the line.

"Everything," I replied, forming my forearms into a mini forklift. Into my arms went books on anatomy and physiology, pathophysiology (the study of disease), advanced cardiac life support, prehospital trauma life support, and our massive main text—Nancy Caroline's *Emergency Care in the Streets*. Often called "the Mother of Paramedics," Nancy Caroline had been the EMS Advisor to President Gerald Ford and she coauthored the first curriculum for paramedics with Dr. Peter Safar in 1974. *Emergency Care in the Streets* quickly became a classic, creating a revolution in the immediate care of the critically ill and injured patients. Before her death in 2002, Caroline recalled her time in prehospital care as among the happiest of her life.

As Mr. Gudger loaded me up with books, my back bent under their weight and I struggled to pull money from my pocket.

"You can pay me later," Mr. Gudger said, laughing at my effort.

As I headed back to the main classroom, I paused in the hall to look again at the class pictures. The oldest photos were in black-and-white and, as the years progressed, the fashion of the times changed from one graduating class to the next. But I saw one similarity—the students all looked supremely confident and competent. I felt another stab of worry. Was I up to the task? Would I succeed? Could I continue their legacy of excellence?

Class 28 had hung a vintage firehouse bell on a plaque as part of their class gift to the school and, just then, Ms. Davis rang it to signal break was over.

After break, Ms. Davis reviewed the course policies. Many were familiar from any academic institution (no cell phone use, no cheating or stealing, no chewing tobacco—though sunflower seeds were acceptable provided no shells ended up on the floor), but a few related specifically to paramedic school and hinted at the challenges ahead. We were to carry a pen, stethoscope, watch, pair of safety glasses, medication guide, and policy manual with us at all times.

"You will be exhausted," Ms. Davis promised us, "but there will be no sleeping in class. However, you can stand in the back of the classroom during lecture if that will help you stay awake."

Each of us was also required to bring "one live person" into school at least once to act as a volunteer patient.

"Kids and parents are especially helpful because they allow us to assess patients with different vital signs and medical histories," she added.

A policy on exposure control dictated what we should do if we were splashed with blood, vomit, or urine during our clinical and field rotations, and the policy regarding "no fighting words" hinted at the paramedic pressure cooker in which we were soon to find ourselves. While we all shared a love of emergency medicine, we were also forty-one type-A personalities who'd be spending virtually every stressful moment for the next four months together. It could get combustible.

At noon, Ms. Davis released us for lunch. I hopped in Wilson's truck along with Lewis, a sponsored firefighter from Santa Monica. Lewis was a tall, athletic guy with a great sense of humor. He could bust into freestyle rap at any moment, and he was a genius at impersonating people. Legend had it he'd even performed some of his proficiency drills during his probationary year as a firefighter in the characters of Robert De Niro and Christopher Walken. We drove down Prairie Avenue, passing the sprawling Inglewood Cemetery, the Forum, and Hollywood Park horse track, and grabbed food at a Taco Bell that had more security than my local bank.

"I'll have a triple steak burrito," I yelled through the bulletproof security glass separating the cashier and kitchen from the dining area. Moments later, the cashier pushed my burrito through a small currency tray.

Outside, a police car blazed by with its sirens blasting and a homeless man haggled for change. *Definitely not New Hampshire,* I thought, taking a bite.

That afternoon, we met our lead lecturer for the classroom portion of paramedic school. "Good afternoon," he began, "I am Mr. Wheeler . . . because no one else wanted to be."

Wilson and I exchanged looks. Was laughing a critical fail criterion in paramedic school?

"The attitude in this room is perfect . . . for a funeral," Mr. Wheeler added with a smirk. "Come on, guys! Lighten up!"

Brian Wheeler was a fiercely intelligent, bespectacled man in his early forties, with a graying beard and a self-deprecating sense of humor. He held an associate of general studies degree and, prior to UCLA, he'd spent years working in Chicago and rural Illinois as a flight paramedic, critical care paramedic, and EMS systems manager. He was also a critical care and pediatric specialist, having taught pediatrics in Europe. With his dry wit and perfect timing, he also happened to be one of the funniest people I've ever met. In short, he was the ideal instructor to keep forty-one action-oriented individuals attentive during four months in the classroom.

Mr. Wheeler began his lecture by speaking about the "awesome responsibility" of being a paramedic and the intense workload of school—"We're going to spoon-feed you with shovels"—but the main point of his lecture concerned teaching us about how to be successful in the program. He spoke about different learning styles—visual, physical, social, and solitary—and offered us effective tips. "Where you study is important," he said, "as is setting up a study schedule, taking breaks, and giving yourself some kind of reward." As he spoke, we all took notes furiously and a dozen digital recorders, placed at the podium, recorded every word.

Most every fire department and ambulance service has a quality assurance (QA) and quality improvement (QI) division and I was glad to find UCLA brought the same mentality to its paramedic program, ensuring the material was presented in various formats—lecture, online, hands-on—to appeal to various learning styles. The school had also studied the correlation between testing time and student success.

"We give you one minute per question," Mr. Wheeler explained. "Any less time is too short; and any more, students tend to overthink questions."

Mr. Wheeler stressed the importance of repetition and an "imitation-practice-precision" model for learning our skills. "Studies have shown it takes between five hundred and one thousand repetitions of a skill to fix it in your muscle memory," he added. During the nine months of school, Mr. Wheeler said, we would endure both critical and cumulative stress and he advised us to eat healthily and get enough sleep and exercise. As he spoke, I decided—given the long hours and constant repetitions of skills—paramedic school would be akin to training for an Olympic event. And the UCLA staff? They'd be like athletic trainers who smile broadly and cheer you on . . . as they're totally kicking your ass.

As five p.m. arrived, Mr. Wheeler advised us to stay on track. "It's a long and difficult track," he explained, "but if you work hard, we believe your success is inevitable and you'll leave here as paramedics."

Patel—the former baker—raised his hand. "What's on the agenda for tomorrow?"

"Tomorrow we begin our tour of the human body," Mr. Wheeler said, shutting off the overhead projector, "and I think you'll find it a very worthwhile trip."

There seemed to be an immediate understanding among everyone in Class 36 that, if we were to pass paramedic school, we would need to come together as a team. So we gathered in the parking lot after class to exchange phone numbers and e-mail addresses and made a pact that we would be one class with one mission.

"I say everyone graduates!" said Miller, a guy from Tennessee with a buzz cut who called all the teachers "ma'am" and "sir."

"That's right!" I added.

"Forty-one students in. Forty-one students out," hollered Carter, a tattooed former Marine who'd recently volunteered with Compton Fire Department.

"Hoo-ah!" yelled O'Brien, the kid, as we all cheered.

We were so naïve.

January

Week One

Private students like myself managed the tuition and high cost of living in L.A. by sharing apartments, living at home with parents, taking out loans, and subsisting on peanut butter and jelly sandwiches. In fact, one student from San Diego, a hulking Samoan named Tilo, planned on sleeping at "Honda Hotel"—his pickup truck—on school nights. On craigslist I found a two-bedroom apartment in El Segundo, which I shared with one roommate, a young engineer in the aerospace industry. The apartment sat on the corner of La Cienega Boulevard and Imperial Highway, in the industrial shadow of LAX; when the planes took off, their engines echoed off the walls.

As I sat down at my desk that first night and cracked open my A & P book, the daunting prospect of school again hit me like a fist. To be honest, a part of me considered fleeing to LAX and departing for some tranquil overseas destination. I could slap the trip on my credit card and arrive by morning. It was a classic fight-or-flight response. But a larger part of myself was ready and eager for the challenge of paramedic school. As I began reading about the organ systems of the body, I realized I was supremely happy out here on the west coast. In Los Angeles, California, among the concrete and palm trees.

The design and function of the human body is one of the most miraculous creations on earth and we began learning about it on the second day of class.

"Who can tell me the definition of disseminated intravascular coagulopathy?" Mr. Wheeler, our lead lecturer, asked us late that afternoon.

None of us knew the answer. As Mr. Wheeler scanned the classroom, I noticed everyone's shoelaces had suddenly become very interesting.

"Anyone? . . . Anyone?" he asked. "Bueller? . . . Bueller?"

We all laughed, recognizing the line from the classic 1980s film, but still no one raised their hand.

Hoping for a better seat at the front of class, I'd arrived at seven thirty on the second day of classes, only to find all the chairs taken once again. Three firefighters from L.A. County had claimed the front row to the right of the podium, and Carter, along with two other Compton Fire Department volunteers, had grabbed the seats to the left. I supposed I could've fought one of them for a seat but, then again, I wasn't really going to try. In the middle of class sat another row of sponsored firefighters—Santa Monica to the left and L.A. County to the right—with private students composing all the remaining rows.

As I looked around that morning, I noticed that even the digital recorders were jockeying for position near the front podium.

Recorders were fanned out around Mr. Wheeler in a wide electronic arc as if he were the president at a press conference. When he took the podium, there was the sound of forty-one notebooks opening and at least a dozen digital recorders clicking on as he prepared to give us a kind of State of the Union on the human body.

It's common knowledge that the fundamental maxim of all health care providers is *Primum non nocere* (Latin for "First, do no harm"). To achieve this, Mr. Wheeler told us, we'd need to have an expert knowledge of the human body, both inside and out. "Topography is important because many of the procedures we perform require you to know specific landmarks on the body to perform them correctly." To start an IV, we needed to differentiate between a vein and an artery. Inserting a breathing tube into the esophagus—which leads to the stomach instead of the lungs— would have dire consequences, and you wouldn't want to mistakenly pierce the heart when you performed a needle decompression to relieve the pressure from a collapsed lung. "This precision is like the difference between a Corvette and a Chevette," Mr. Wheeler quipped.

We also needed to know the levels of organization found within the body—chemicals, cells, tissues, organs—and the ten organ systems such as the cardiac, respiratory, skeletal, and nervous system. "These organ systems all work together to form *homeostasis*," Mr. Wheeler explained, "a condition when the many variables of the body are controlled so internal conditions remain stable and constant." How do our bodies achieve this? We shiver, or sweat, to maintain an internal temperature around 98.6 degrees. Clots form in a laceration to stop the bleeding, and the swelling around a sprained ankle forms a natural cast. Baroreceptors in the arteries, sensing a drop in the blood flow of the body, signal the sympathetic nervous system to increase heart rate and constrict vessels to raise blood pressure. And, when they sense an increase in arterial carbon dioxide and a decrease in oxygen, chemoreceptors in the brain signal respiratory muscles to breathe deeper and faster.

"The body is a stacked system, which is good," Mr. Wheeler explained, "but it also has more opportunity to break down."

Along with a stable temperature, human homeostasis also depend on acid/base balance in the arterial blood pH between 7.35 and 7.45. How is this achieved? A delicate buffer system of proteins, bicarbonate, and phosphate ions usually maintain this balance but it could easily be disrupted, severely affecting both metabolism and respiratory status. The goal of all the interventions we performed as paramedics—administering oxygen, IV fluids, and medications— was to restore homeostasis in a human body that was slow, or no longer able, to do so.

To start us thinking critically, Mr. Wheeler gave us the example of a heroin addict found unresponsive in an alley. "Would this patient initially be suffering from respiratory acidosis or alkalosis?"

A hand shot up from the center of the room. It was Lewis, the firefighter from Santa Monica. "Respiratory acidosis," he said. "Heroin is a central nervous system depressant so the patient's respiratory rate would be low, causing an acid buildup."

"Good," said Mr. Wheeler, nodding. "What about a woman having a panic attack and hyperventilating?"

Miller raised his hand. "Well, sir, she'd be breathing really fast and shallow so she'd likely be suffering from respiratory alkalosis," he said with a southern drawl.

Mr. Wheeler agreed. "That patient thinks she needs oxygen but what she really needs is more carbon dioxide to even out the pH."

Metabolic alkalosis was rare, but we'd often encounter meta- bolic acidosis—when oxygen-starved cells in the body produced lactic acid—with patients in shock and cardiac arrest. Mr. Wheeler informed us that a small change of 0.1 in either the acidotic or alkalotic direction from the normal 7.35–7.45 balance could send our patient on a roller-coaster ride toward shock, coma, and death . . . and that's where we came in.

That afternoon, Mr. Wheeler lectured on medical terminology. Medical terminology uses root words, prefixes, and suffixes to describe components, conditions, and processes in the human body and is supposed to help ease communication between health care professionals, though it certainly didn't feel like it. I couldn't understand how referring to a bloody nose as an *epistaxis* had any value whatsoever, but I was soon to learn otherwise.

It was like studying a new language as Mr. Wheeler introduced us to terms like *hematuria* (blood in the urine) and *petechiae* (purple spots on the body). We would now refer to "front" and "back" as *anterior* and *posterior*. "Closest to" and "farther away" would now be known as *proximal* and *distal*, and *superior* and *inferior* would replace "above" and "below." With a sly grin, Mr. Wheeler informed us that many terms we'd once used would no longer work. "Adam's apple" would be replaced with *thyroid cartilage*. *Calcaneal tendon* would substitute for "Achilles tendon," and suddenly our thoracic cavities were filled with—who knew!—*true*, *false*, and *floating ribs*. Evidently, there were also invisible planes in our bodies, slicing them from front to back (*frontal plane*), top to bottom (*horizontal plane*), and right to left (*median plane*). Perhaps the tension I was feeling at the abundance of the material was *eustress*— the good kind of stress that motivates you to keep working—but good God if it didn't feel a lot more like *distress*.

Despite the abundance of new and unfamiliar words, Mr. Wheeler assured us we could learn medicine by learning medical terminology. For instance, on a 911 call, we'd not always know or have the time to look up every medical condition our patients had, but we could figure them out by using our knowledge of medical terminology.

"Let's start with *disseminated*," he said. "Can anyone venture a guess?"

I raised my hand in class for the first time. I recalled the word from an SAT prep class. "*Disseminated* means spread out widely," I said.

Mr. Wheeler nodded. "What about *inter*?" he then asked.

"Inside," said a student named Jones, a quiet guy from Redondo Beach and a recent USC grad.

"Good! And *vascular*?"

O'Brien's hand shot up with youthful enthusiasm. "Something having to do with a vein."

Carter waved a tattooed arm and reminded us that *coagulation* concerned the process of clotting, and we all recalled that -*pathy* denoted a disorder with a particular part of the body.

"Now who can put the phrase together?" Mr. Wheeler asked about *disseminated intravascular coagulopathy*.

After thinking for a moment, Fowler, the one female in our class, raised her hand. She'd grown up in San Bernardino and had worked as an EMT at the Coachella and Stagecoach music festivals prior to paramedic school. She drove a large white pickup truck with a light bar on top and liked to shoot guns on her days off. "The widespread inability to clot inside a vein," she ventured.

"Exactly," Mr. Wheeler said, proudly. "See how well this works?"

Before we left, Mr. Wheeler gave us our first homework assignment. By Thursday, we needed to read the first chapter of *Emergency Care in the Streets*, the first chapter and all the appendixes of our anatomy and physiology book, watch an online video on the history of EMS, and prepare for our first quiz, which would cover medical terminology and the organization of the body.

Miller raised his hand and politely asked how disseminated intravascular coagulopathy would present in the field.

Mr. Wheeler said we'd know it when we saw it. "Your patient would be circling the drain and bleeding from every orifice."

"How do you treat that?" I asked.

Mr. Wheeler smiled. "Drive fast."

Before classes had started, I'd pledged that I would try to treat myself with the same level of care during paramedic school that I would extend to patients. I vowed to keep a regular exercise schedule, eat healthily, and make an effort to maintain a normal sleep schedule. I also planned to keep a journal in which I'd record daily thoughts, observations, and, if needed, any "fighting words." We hadn't even had our first quiz and already I felt the first stage of the stress response: alarm. Historically, the alarm response was beneficial—it poised our ancestors for attack and helped them outrun predators—but I knew it would be unhealthy if it continued. So on our first day off of classes, I slept until nine and started my day with a run at the beach; grabbed coffee; and then hit the grocery store to buy some healthy food.

Sounds good, right?

Bad idea.

I didn't crack open a book until two p.m., at which point the amount of material I needed to know for the quiz slapped me with a textbook-sized fist. The first chapters of *Emergency Care in the Streets* and our A & P book weren't too bad—what overwhelmed me was the 170 abbreviations, forty medical terms, and dozens of prefixes, suffixes, and units of measurement I had to learn for my first quiz the following day. The terms weren't easy, either, and abbreviations like GFR and HLA stood for *glomerular filtration rate* (a kidney test) and the *human leukocyte antigen* (a gene essential to the immune system) weren't exactly no-brainers.

I made a fresh pot of coffee, tore open a thick stack of white flash cards, and immediately began writing. Four hours later, when I'd made only a modest dent in the material, it dawned on me that I was

spending all my time creating flash cards and none of my time studying them. I tossed the note cards aside and decided to read terms
aloud, hoping that would drill them into my memory. By eleven p.m.
I was exhausted, so I decided to take a study break. Except, in paramedic school, a "study break" doesn't mean you stop working—it
just means that you switch to studying something else.

I powered up my computer and clicked on the video we'd been
assigned to watch about the history of modern EMS in America.
A railway man named Julian Stanley Wise created the first volunteer ambulance service in Virginia, the Roanoke Life Saving and
First Aid Crew, in 1928. When Wise was a boy, he'd watched helplessly as two men flipped their canoe and drowned in the Roanoke
River. "Right then, I resolved that I was going to become a lifesaver.
Never again would I watch a man die when he could be saved," he
would later say. When news of his rescue squad's success spread,
similar units sprang up around the rest of the country. Later, when
World War II drained hospital staff, emergency care increasingly
began to fall on volunteers—but despite good intentions, these
volunteers often responded to accidents with little training and poor
equipment.

In 1966, the National Academy of Sciences published a white
paper titled "Accidental Death and Disability: The Neglected Disease of Modern Society." The report cited traumatic injury as the
number one cause of death in Americans between one and thirty-
seven years old. It also declared the lack of a comprehensive EMS
system to be America's "most important environmental health
problem" and found that the chances of survival for a person who
was seriously injured in the United States "would be better in a zone
of combat than on the average city street."

Congress and President Lyndon Johnson responded by signing
the National Highway Safety Act into legislation, which dictated
minimum standards for ambulance design, equipment, and the

attendants who treated patients. The white paper also initiated a number of paramedic pilot programs across the country, in Miami, L.A., and Seattle. By 1970, while many Americans were still focused on space and Neil Armstrong's historic walk on the moon, an equally impressive miracle was taking place back on earth— paramedics were waking people up from the dead.

By eight a.m. the next day, I was seated in the main classroom of the Walter S. Graf Center with a #2 pencil in my hand and a multiple choice quiz and Scantron sheet in front of me.

I'd arrived at 7:20 that morning but was again relegated to a seat in the far back. Frustrated, I sought out Michael Gudger, the registration coordinator, for some inside information regarding arrival times. "They're waiting for me when I get here at seven," he said with the mild dismay of every worker who has to show a public face before their first cup of coffee.

Disheartened and sleep deprived, I sat next to Wilson, who mentioned forgoing a surf on his day off in favor of studying. I pulled out my A & P book and flipped through the pages but couldn't concentrate. The anxiety in the room could've lit a power station. O'Brien was incessantly tapping his foot with a teenager's attention span. Patel, the baker, chomped loudly on gum. Miller tapped his pencil nervously, while Carter and Lewis were reviewing note cards out loud, with Lewis occasionally answering as Christopher Walken. My coffee buzz was wearing off and the lack of sleep was quickly catching up with me. I was crashing right before the quiz.

At eight o'clock, Mr. Wheeler handed out our quiz materials. "Fill in all bubbles completely and thoroughly erase all mistakes," he said. "You have forty-five minutes."

There was a lot riding on this first quiz. Everyone in Class 36 wanted to get off on the right foot and take the lead in the race for valedictorian. Maybe the quiz would be inconsequential in the grand scheme of things, but that morning, it felt like a predictor of success for the entire paramedic program. But if the first few questions were any indication . . . I was in trouble. Did the *mesentery* or *peritoneum* cover the abdominal organs? What was the difference between *parietal* and *visceral* pain? What did the suffix *-poiesis* mean? Was pregnancy a positive feedback mechanism? And what the hell was the *loop of Henle*? It sounded like the lead singer of the Eagles—and right then, paramedic school sure felt like Hotel California, which at first seemed so alluring until you discovered it was really a prison.

I skipped the questions I didn't know, vowing to return to them, and continued on in the quiz. To my great relief, I nailed the next three questions, before getting tripped up on the definition of *gluconeogenesis*; then I remembered how Mr. Wheeler had instructed us to break the term down using medical terminology. I knew the word *gluco* related to sugar. *Neo* meant new, or young. And I recalled from church that *genesis* involved creation or formation. The definition, "the generation of glucose from noncarbohydrate substrates," suddenly seemed obvious. I hit my stride after that, and the rest of the quiz questions blazed by in a blur.

"Five minutes," Mr. Wheeler announced, gazing at the clock.

I raced through the remaining questions, then went back to answer the ones I'd left blank. I took some educated guesses, figuring it was better than leaving them blank.

"Time!" Mr. Wheeler said. "Put your pencils down."

We reviewed the quiz for a half hour after we handed our sheets in. Mr. Wheeler would read a question out loud and one of us would raise a hand to answer. A lot of the questions were ambiguous by design. "We believe the discussion a question generates is equally important as the answer," Mr. Wheeler said. "Our goal is to create critical thinkers, not 'monkey see, monkey do' medics."

He spent the remainder of the morning lecturing on the chemistry of life—hydrogen bonds, ionic bonds, covalent bonds—and, in the afternoon, we met another instructor, Nanci Medina, for the first time.

"You can call me Mrs. Medina or Sarge," she explained. "And I apologize in advance if any swearwords slip out of my mouth."

Mrs. Medina, a peppy, blond woman in her late forties, was herself a graduate of the Daniel Freeman paramedic school and had worked for years with L.A. County Sheriff's Department as an undercover agent and retired as a sergeant detective. She'd received her bachelor's in EMS and now worked part-time as a paramedic with the Sierra Madre Fire Department. Along with lecturing, Mrs. Medina would be the one who assigned us to our clinical rotations and internship spots.

"A good person to know," I whispered to Wilson.

Naturally, we used any opportunity to ask about field internships, the one aspect of paramedic school that worried all of us the most.

Mrs. Medina didn't sugarcoat it. She said she'd seen more men cry during field internship than anywhere else. "And that includes funerals," she added. "That's why I keep a box of tissues on my desk."

There was a Ping-Pong table in one of the spare rooms at school and, during breaks, it was quickly becoming our favorite gathering place—a chance to whack away all the stress and tension by inflicting harm on a little yellow plastic ball. That afternoon, Miller and Lewis were in the midst of a spirited game of doubles with me and O'Brien—the oldest student paired with the youngest—but when Mr. Gudger strolled past with our quiz grades, we dropped our paddles and joined the stampede of students following him.

"Patience, guys," Mr. Gudger said as we filed in behind him, "patience."

Mr. Gudger posted the grades on a glass-enclosed bulletin board at the far end of the main hallway and we quickly huddled around. The top of the sheet reminded us of the strict grading criteria for paramedic school: A > 93 percent, B > 85 percent, C > 80 percent. D grades didn't exist. And anything less than 79 percent meant failure. Our class numbers were listed immediately below with our grade.

"Nailed it," exclaimed Carter, high-fiving Lewis so hard it echoed off the walls.

"Ninety-four percent!" added Patel.

"I feel the need . . . the need for speed," said Miller, quoting the movie *Top Gun*. He'd scored 90 percent.

Other students weren't so fortunate.

"Missed it by five points," said Tilo, his hulking figure deflating with worry.

Jones, the quiet USC grad, dropped his head when he saw his score and skulked away.

When I arrived at the bulletin board, I discovered I'd answered thirty-seven out of forty-three questions correct, earning 86 percent. "Sweet!" I exclaimed, giving O'Brien a high five.

I was thrilled . . . but my excitement was short-lived. As I walked away, it dawned on me that my score was one of the lowest in the class, and I had been only seven points away from failing.

January

BSI . . . Scene Safe

As the first week of classes came to a close, we learned about patient assessment, the foundation of everything paramedics did.

"Every assessment begins with taking body substance isolation and ensuring scene safety," said Justin McCullough, pointing to a patient flowchart on the PowerPoint presentation.

Mr. McCullough was an enthusiastic man in his mid-thirties with so much energy you'd think he had Red Bull instead of blood coursing through his veins. Prior to teaching, he'd graduated from Daniel Freeman and was the first student ever awarded the Clinical Excellence Award for patient care. He worked for the Los Angeles Fire Department, was injured on duty, but continues to work as a paramedic during NASCAR events at the Auto Club Speedway in Fontana.

At the words "body substance isolation" and "scene safety," the class emitted a collective groan. These were both topics that had already been drilled into us since our first day of EMT class, long before paramedic school, and, frankly, we were all sick of it.

"Not taking or verbalizing BSI and scene safety is a critical fail on every skill," Mr. McCullough said. "So I suggest you do."

Our first day of patient assessment began with Mr. McCullough dividing the class up into teams of six students each (and one group of five), mirroring how, on many 911 calls, the fire department responds with an ambulance staffed by two paramedics and a fire engine of four firefighters who assist with patient care, movement, extrication, interviewing bystanders, crowd control, or documentation. Our teams would remain a unit for the length of the course and were meant to teach us how to be both good team leaders and good team members. I was assigned to Team 3 with Miller, O'Brien, Jones, Carter, and Lewis, who, when Mr. McCullough called his name, responded as Robert De Niro in *Taxi Driver*, asking, "You talkin' to me?" Along with practicing skills as a team, we would also handle "station duties" at school, such as emptying the trash and taking out the recycling.

In addition to the two main classrooms—with their traditional podium and desk layout—the Walter S. Graf Center also had a kitchen, a computer room, and twenty scenario rooms in which we'd practice our skills. Some rooms had only a table and a few chairs scattered about. Other rooms were staged with furniture: scenario room 5 had a couch and TV, like a living room; scenario room 6 had a hospital bed, IV pole, and machine for taking vital signs, like an ER; and scenario room 7 was a nursery with a cradle and stuffed animals. I felt a little sad even walking past that one.

Our equipment lockers lined the far wall of scenario room 1. There were seven lockers, each bearing a number and color designation. Team 3's color was yellow. Our locker was stuffed with a cardiac monitor, a blue "first-in" medication bag, a green airway bag, and an orange trauma box. Our first task was to do inventory and make sure our locker had all of our equipment. Mr. McCullough handed each group an inventory list for each piece of equipment. It was detailed, right down to the number of tiny alcohol prep pads.

"I want you to pull out everything and make sure all the equipment is there," he instructed. "Forgetting a piece of equipment during a practical skills test is just as bad as showing up on scene empty-handed."

I grabbed the cardiac monitor. O'Brien threw the airway bag over his shoulder and Miller and Carter took the first-in bag and trauma box. We assembled in scenario room 15, which was empty except for a gurney and a large black file cabinet. As I opened the cabinet up, a plastic baby head tumbled out. I jumped back in surprise. At times, paramedic school felt like a House of Horrors—you never knew what creepy lifelike item you'd find when you opened a door or cabinet. It might be a rubber arm on which we'd perform IVs, or a man's head to practice intubation, or a female's pelvis for OB skills. Many of the mannequins had funny names like Airway Adam or Megacode Carl, but they could be truly unnerving.

We pulled out all our equipment, emptying each pocket, and, when we finished, every inch of the floor in scenario room 15 was covered with medication vials, breathing tubes, bags of IV fluid, oxygen masks, rolls of gauze, trauma dressings, ECG electrodes, carbon dioxide detectors, tourniquets, and much more. Looking at all the equipment, it seemed impossible we would learn both how—and when—to use everything in a medical emergency. "An awesome responsibility," Mr. Wheeler, our lead lecturer, had said, and I was beginning to see why.

After sorting through all the gear and confirming that everything was there, we returned it to our locker and reconvened in the main classroom, where Mr. McCullough, our skills coordinator, displayed a patient assessment flowchart. As many of us were already aware, most of the scene size-up took place even before we stepped out of the ambulance. Once we'd sized up the scene and donned personal protective equipment such as exam gloves and safety glasses, we'd begin the primary assessment of our patient.

"What things are we looking for with our general impression?" Mr. McCullough asked.

O'Brien shot his hand up. "The patient's appearance. Their work of breathing and position."

"Exactly," Mr. McCullough replied. "A call where a patient is lying facedown is totally different from one where someone is up and talking with you."

We determined a patient's level of responsiveness by assessing if he or she was alert and conscious. We'd ask patients to state their names, and if they knew the date and where they were, to see if they were also oriented. If so, we'd then ask the patient why 911 had been called. On the other hand, if a patient wasn't responsive upon our arrival, we'd attempt to rouse him using our voice or a painful stimulus such as pressing firmly on a fingernail bed. If we were unable to wake him, we'd assume he was unconscious, and continue with our assessment.

After determining responsiveness, we moved on to the ABCs: airway, breathing, and circulation. If the patient was speaking to us, we could reasonably assume that he or she had an open airway. But in other cases, we might need to remove broken teeth, blood, or vomit from the patient's airway using a suction device, or insert something such as an oropharyngeal airway (OPA), a curved plastic device that prevents the tongue from covering the windpipe.

"As you move through your primary assessment, you treat problems as you find them," Mr. McCullough instructed. "You don't move on until you fix it." He clarified that we weren't actually counting the pulse or number of respirations or getting a full set of vital signs during the primary assessment. "Will taking someone's vital signs save their life?" he asked rhetorically. "No. The purpose of checking the airway, breathing, and circulation is to quickly determine—and treat—any immediate life threats."

Once the airway was clear, we'd assess the rate, rhythm, and quality of breathing.

Miller raised his hand and said, "We can also listen to lung sounds, sir. See if they have any wheezes or fluid in there."

Lewis added that we could also treat injuries that were causing compromised breathing, such as performing a needle decompression, which involved inserting a catheter into the chest wall to relieve a tension pneumothorax, a buildup of pressure in the lungs that sometimes occurred after a penetrating or blunt injury.

Mr. McCullough nodded, then moved on. "So your patient has an unobstructed airway; you've assessed breathing and have them on oxygen. How do we assess circulation?"

Jones raised his hand. I was surprised—he'd hardly said a word since class began, but he nailed the answer. "We assess if the pulse is weak or strong, regular or irregular," he began. "We also check the patient's skin signs for color, temperature, and moisture. Manage any life-threatening bleeding and, if indicated, treat for shock."

After the ABCs, the next thing to assess was the size and reactivity of a patient's pupils—which could clue in paramedics to a stroke, skull fracture, or narcotic overdose—and check for any abnormal positioning of the patient's arms and legs, such as being rigidly flexed, which might suggest a spinal injury.

"Once we have all this information, how do we make a transport decision?" Mr. McCullough asked the class.

Fowler raised her hand. "If there's no major deficit to the ABCs, you have time to stay on scene and perform your secondary assessment."

"Exactly," said Mr. McCullough, clicking off the projector. "You have time to obtain vital signs and find out about the patient's medical history, allergies, and medications."

And if the patient didn't pass the assessments?

"We'd want to be off scene and en route to the hospital in ten minutes," Carter stated, raising his hand. "Code 3. Lights and sirens."

After a weekend that passed in the blink of an eye (and a heavy-duty study load), Monday picked up with Ms. Davis, the program director, lecturing us on the steps for a secondary assessment.

"The secondary assessment forms the bottom half of our flow-chart and begins after we've checked ABCs and made a transport decision," Ms. Davis had told us earlier that day. "If the patient is critical, you perform the secondary assessment en route to the hospital. If the patient is stable, you can complete it on scene."

The secondary assessment consisted of performing a physical exam; taking a set of vital signs (pulse, respiratory rate, blood pressure, temperature [if indicated] and assessing the patient's level of pain); and other diagnostic tests such as checking a patient's ECG, blood sugar, and the amount of oxygen in his or her blood (pulse oximetry). We'd also inquire about the patient's medical history, ask specific questions about the illness or injury, formulate a treatment and transport plan, and reassess the patient and success of our interventions.

Most of the patient assessment was similar to what I'd learned in EMT class, but as paramedics, we would take a leadership role on the calls, delegating jobs such as measuring vital signs and spinal immobilization to the other members of our crew. For example, as an EMT, if a patient complained of chest pain, I had two courses of action—call for paramedics or transport the patient rapidly to the hospital. Now, as a paramedic, I'd have the ability to investigate the *nature* of the chest pain and decide if it was cardiac related, a case of pneumonia, pulmonary embolism (a clot in the lungs), trauma, or emotional upset, and treat it accordingly.

As with everything else we'd learn in paramedic school, there was an art to acquiring information on scene. "Ask open-ended questions instead of ones with simple yes or no answers," Ms. Davis advised. "The goal is to keep the patient talking about their condition and obtain key information."

She coached us on using interview techniques to facilitate effective communication. *Repeating* key words kept patients focused and prompted them to continue talking. *Clarification* encouraged patients to delve deeper into certain answers; *confrontation* pointed out something interesting in patients' behavior; while using a phrase like "please go on" lets patients know you understood their complaint.

Ms. Davis split up the class into pairs and we practiced using the interview techniques on each other. Then she asked for two volunteers to demonstrate at the front of the class. Lewis immediately stood.

"I'll do it," he said, "but only if I can be the patient."

"Sure," Ms. Davis replied, knowing we were in for a show.

As he made his way to the front, Lewis grabbed a blanket from one of the cabinets and threw it over his head, morphing into the kind of homeless man we'd all seen on L.A. street corners.

Carter leapt up to play the paramedic role, and as he approached Lewis, the firefighter grew more agitated, shifting in his seat and looking over his shoulder.

"Help!" he yelled. "They're everywhere!"

"Hello, sir," Carter said. "What seems to be the problem today?"

"I see dead people!" Lewis yelled, shaking.

We all busted up, recalling the classic scene from the movie *The Sixth Sense*.

"You see dead people?" Carter asked seriously, kneeling next to him.

"Everywhere," Lewis replied, swatting the air. "They're trying to catch me!"

As Lewis grew more anxious, our laughter grew louder.

"Please go on," said Carter, fixing his gaze on Lewis.

But as we realized Lewis and Carter weren't joking around, our chuckles quickly died down.

"They've been after me for two days," Lewis replied from under his blanket.

Carter put a hand on Lewis's shoulder and told him that was understandable. "I am here for you and I'm not going to leave your side until we get to the hospital."

The room was quiet by now. We were all riveted. There was something real going on here. It wasn't just the arrival of a paramedic, but the arrival of hope, support, and someone willing to give a scared man some time.

When Carter asked Lewis if he had any plans to hurt himself or others, Lewis shook his head no, then peeked out of the blanket.

"Do you see dead people?" Lewis asked Carter, shaking less now and delivering an Academy Award–worthy performance.

Carter said he didn't. "But I'm sure they look real to you . . ."

When Carter obtained his patient history, Lewis revealed that the character he was playing had a history of paranoid schizophrenia and hadn't been taking his meds.

"When was the last time you took your meds?" Carter asked to clarify.

"Two days ago."

"Was that about the time the dead people started appearing?" Lewis nodded.

"Can I take you to the hospital to get checked out?" Carter asked, offering a hand.

Lewis calmly stood. "Okay, but you won't let the dead people hurt me?"

"I promise we'll take great care of you," Carter assured him.

Carter walked Lewis out the side door, and we all burst into wild applause.

The following afternoon, Baxter Larmon gave his first lecture. Dr. Larmon was director of the UCLA Center for Prehospital Care and a professor of medicine at the UCLA School of Medicine. He had a PhD and more than forty years of experience in EMS, had spoken at hundreds of conferences, written more than sixty publications in emergency medicine, won lifetime achievement awards, and was named one of the most influential people in the profession by the *Journal of Emergency Medicine Services.*

Dr. Larmon lectured us on the art of patient assessment and encouraged us to use all of our senses when treating a patient, including scent. "You will learn to smell death," he told us. "You'll be able to walk into a house and say, 'There's a dead person in here.'" Like the wise elder he was, imparting his knowledge on us new initiates, Dr. Larmon spoke about the necessity of staying calm amid chaos on scene, of finding the "flow" of the call. "You need to learn what normal is so you can spot abnormal," he said. "You may not know exactly what abnormal is, but you'll know it's not normal."

A few days later was our first day of skills training, where we'd start putting more and more of what we were hearing in the classroom to practice. We'd perform tasks like obtaining patient histories, listening to lung sounds, performing physical assessments, and checking finger stick blood glucose tests. The skills instructors taught us using a principle known as "whole-part-whole." They'd begin by demonstrating the skill in its entirety, then spend a few minutes breaking it apart into each individual step. When they finished, they'd demonstrate it again, and then release us to practice. Each practical skills session lasted about an hour and, near the end of it, one of our classmates performed the skill for the group. In my group, Team 3, Carter had demonstrated the detailed assessment during our first session, in scenario room 2—"I'm palpating the four quadrants of the abdomen for any rigidity, rebound tenderness, pulsating masses, distention, or discoloration"—and then, in scenario room 15, Jones took a comprehensive patient history from O'Brien, who was posing as a high school student with abdominal pain.

"You're up, Grange," O'Brien said now, pointing to the center of the room. "Show us what you've got!"

We were in scenario room 14, which was lined with IV poles with bags of normal saline hanging off them and a table full of medications, catheters, and tiny blue IV tourniquets. The far end of the table had been cleared for the blood glucose skill. A mannequin arm lay atop a blue "chux" absorbent pad, next to which sat alcohol prep pads, lancets, test strips, and a glucometer.

I pulled on a pair of blue exam gloves, set my safety goggles on my nose, and wrapped a stethoscope over my shoulders. "To begin, I'd like to explain what kinds of patients need a blood sugar check," I said, addressing my team and the instructor. "Diabetic patients, but also people feeling dizzy, weak, who are altered, or who've had a seizure."

I approached the table. "The first thing I'm going to do is grab my alcohol prep pad—"

Greg Hurley, our skills instructor, quickly cut me off. "Don't forget to say 'BSI' and 'scene safe,'" he reminded me. Mr. Hurley was a retired firefighter/paramedic who also taught advanced cardiac life support classes.

I nodded and walked back to the door to start over. "First thing I'm going to do is take BSI and ensure my scene is safe," I said.

"Your scene is safe," Mr. Hurley replied.

I quickly verbalized the indications for taking a blood sugar sample and then approached the IV arm. It was ashen gray with ropy veins that had been poked and prodded so many times by paramedic students, I actually felt bad for it.

I grabbed an alcohol prep pad to swab a finger.

"Which hand are you using?" Mr. Hurley asked.

My right, I told him.

"Is your patient right or left handed?"

I shrugged my shoulders. "Not sure."

"Try to use their nondominant hand," Mr. Hurley announced, before asking me to continue. "It's less invasive."

I tore open the alcohol prep pad and swabbed the side of the thumb. As I did, Mr. Hurley asked me to verbalize why I'd picked that location. "During a skill, I need to not only see what you're doing but also hear what you're thinking," he said.

"I'm wiping the side of the finger to cleanse the site, and I'm using the side of the finger because it hurts less," I replied.

"Good," he said. "Continue."

I grabbed the lancet. "And now I'm going to puncture the skin to obtain a blood sample."

Before I could, Mr. Hurley stopped me once again. "Did you wait until the alcohol dried?" he asked. "If not, it will prevent the blood from forming a well-rounded drop and might ruin the sample."

I fanned the mannequin's finger, feeling the weight of my teammates' eyes on me. When they'd demonstrated their skills, it had been fluid and effortless, and the other instructors had only stopped them every few steps. *Am I screwing up?* The actual process of testing blood sugar wasn't hard—just poke the skin and collect the blood—but proficiency in paramedic school demanded that we break every skill down into the smallest steps, and verbalize everything, which I was having trouble remembering to do.

"Once the finger is dry, I will obtain my blood sample," I said, using the small plastic lancet to make a tiny puncture. "And then

I will dispose of my lancet in the sharps container," I said, placing it into a red plastic container.

"Next I'm going to squeeze the finger to attain a drop of blood," I continued. The mannequin arm didn't actually bleed (thank God), but I simulated it lightly, and touched the "blood" with a test strip, which I then placed in the glucometer machine.

"What are you doing while you're waiting for a reading?" Mr. Hurley asked.

I wasn't sure, but looked up to see my teammate O'Brien motion to his finger.

"I'm going to wipe the remaining blood from the finger and apply pressure until the bleeding stops," I said quickly. Next, I simulated placing a Band-Aid over the site. "And last, I will dispose of my equipment in an aseptic manner and reassess my patient."

Mr. Hurley asked what a normal blood sugar reading would be.

I blanked. Once again, I felt the weight of everyone's eyes on me. "Between 60 and 100," I ventured.

"Eighty and 120," Mr. Hurley corrected me.

Just then, Mr. McCullough rang the firehouse bell in the hallway, signaling it was time to switch skills.

"Decent job," Mr. Hurley said. "Keep practicing."

I quickly gathered my things, unhappy with my performance. My skill had been full of fumbling and there was no flow to it. If I couldn't perform a simple finger stick easily, how could I hope to master a skill like intubation, which had twenty-two different steps?

"Keep your head up," said Carter, with a slap on the back that sent me stumbling forward. "It's early in the game."

Martin Luther King Jr. Day gave us a three-day weekend before our third week of classes, but all it really meant was that we didn't get our usual Wednesday off and instead had four straight days of class. That Thursday, defense attorney David Givot spoke to our class about professional liability. Mr. Givot was a fellow Daniel Freeman graduate who'd worked in the field as a paramedic for a few years before attending law school with the hope of representing EMS providers throughout the country.

He emphasized the enormous responsibility we were undertaking. "Someone is going to put their life entirely into your hands, and if you're not up for it, there's the door!" he said, pointing.

As paramedics, we would practice medicine and save lives in every kind of environment—in crowded bars, in dark alleys, on the sides of highways—and we'd work long hours, in heat, rain, snow, and sleet. And we'd also operate under the constant threat of lawsuits.

Certainly some lawsuits were valid and fair. But some were questionable, like when a family sued the City of Los Angeles because LAFD paramedics refused to enter the scene of a shooting until the police arrived and determined the area safe. Then there was the case of a man in Nevada who'd died of a heart attack, and his family sued the paramedics for being delayed at an unmanned security gate outside his apartment complex. But perhaps the most distressing lawsuit occurred in Florida in 2010. A woman had given birth in an ambulance during transport from one hospital to another. The baby was born breach, fifteen weeks premature, and without a pulse. Miraculously, the paramedics brought the baby back to life, only to have their ambulance service sued for $10 million. The reason? The baby was born with some birth defects and the family thought the paramedics should have refused a direct order from the physician and not transported the pregnant mother in the first place. Despite the paramedics' incredible field save, the jury sided with the plaintiff, awarding a $10 million professional negligence suit against the ambulance service.

Mr. Givot reminded us that people call 911 because they're in over their heads, or they *feel* that they're in over their heads. "And yet, the fastest, most unpredictable twist of fate can cost you everything. Every step through the criminal system has a direct effect on our license, livelihood, and life," he said.

Mr. Givot lectured on the justice system and how it related specifically to EMS. "Where most people deal in dollars, you deal in people's lives." Along with being held liable for negligence (failure to exercise appropriate care), we could also be liable for nonfeasance (failure to perform), misfeasance (intentionally performing a harmful and injurious act), and, of course, compromising patient privacy by posting a comment or image on social media. At the same time, however, the largest number of lawsuits actually concerned ambulance collisions.

Fowler, the woman with the big pickup truck, raised her hand. "How do you avoid liability?"

Mr. Givot's answer sounded a lot like our earlier lectures on good patient care. "Perform a thorough assessment on each and every patient. Provide treatment that is within your scope of practice, and document everything," he advised. "Nothing is more important than the patient you're with."

"If you didn't document it, you didn't do it," repeated Wilson, who'd somehow managed to squeeze in a surf session on our day off.

"So who's going to walk out?" Mr. Givot asked, glancing at the door—the door that led to the hallway, which led to the exit, which led to the parking lot, which led to dozens of less stressful careers. "There is absolutely no shame in saying, 'This is not the profession for me,' and walking out."

His lecture had introduced us to a reality about the paramedic profession that many of us hadn't contemplated before. A moment of truth had arrived for every student in the room.

"There's no shame in not finishing paramedic school," Mr. Givot said again.

And who from Class 36 walked out the door? Not one of us even glanced at it.

The following morning, just after eight, we had some unexpected excitement in the form of paramedics from the L.A. County Fire Department in Inglewood getting dispatched to our UCLA paramedic school for a student with chest pain.

While it might've been normal for our hearts to start racing the moment we turned onto Grace Street and approached campus, Patel didn't just feel his heart racing that day—and it wasn't that pecan-crusted chicken he'd baked the night before, either—instead, he said, he felt a pressure at the center of his chest as if someone were sitting on it.

"Unprovoked. A two out of ten in severity and nonradiating," Patel told Ms. Davis, who probably never thought she'd be taking a patient history on a student.

As Patel spoke with Ms. Davis, his chest pressure diminished, but school policy required he be assessed by paramedics anyway. When the fire department paramedics arrived on scene, they performed a full workup on Patel—obtained vital signs, did a 12-lead ECG, and took his pulse oximetry. The lead medic had graduated from UCLA a few years prior. As he hopped off the truck and approached Patel, the paramedic raised his hands and said to Ms. Davis, "At this time I am going to take full BSI precautions and ensure my scene is safe."

"Your scene is safe," Patel said, laughing.

Patel declined transport to the hospital and returned to the main classroom for our morning lecture. Maybe his pain was unprovoked—

or maybe he'd just realized that our first block exam was on Monday.

Our first block exam covered patient assessment and EMS systems. EMS systems concerned topics such as the varying types of ambulances, licenses, certifications, and radio wavelengths, and the difference between expressed and implied consent (i.e., consent given verbally versus that which one assumed a patient would give if he or she were alert and oriented).

I'd studied until two a.m. for the block, at which point I'd collapsed into bed exhausted, my body desperate for sleep . . . although it took almost another two hours for my brain to get the message. I drifted off around four, and when my alarm went off at five thirty, I awoke with a violent start.

Despite my lack of sleep, I found myself well prepared as I filled in ovals on the Scantron for my first block exam. Yet this confidence felt more worrisome than the dread and anxiety I usually felt when taking a quiz. Had I answered the questions too fast? Missed key information? I finished the block with twenty minutes remaining and used the extra time to review my answers.

The moment time was up on the block exam, we handed them in and plunged right into Mr. Wheeler's famed "Airway Academy," where we'd learn skills to manage a patient's airway—that ever-important "A" of the patient assessment ABCs. Over the next ten days, we'd be quizzed on every structure of the trachea and the glottic opening, and we'd practice our first paramedic-level intervention: intubation, the process of inserting a breathing tube into a patient's windpipe.

"You don't try to get an airway, you *get* an airway," Mr. Wheeler said as he put a picture of the glottic opening on the overhead projector. "If you don't have an airway, you have nothing."

Patients in respiratory or cardiac arrest—or who were unconscious and without a gag reflex—couldn't protect their airways, so intubation corrected that critical problem. If done correctly, intubation prevented fluid, like blood or vomit, from entering the lungs, and it also allowed tracheal suctioning and decreased gastric inflation—which could compress major vessels, causing a decrease in blood pressure—and offered another way to deliver medications if you couldn't use an IV. Intubation had other benefits, too, such as facilitating continuous chest compressions during CPR and reducing anatomical "dead space"—the portion of the respiratory tract from the mouth to the lungs where air tends to sit and grow stale instead of participating in the exchange of oxygen and carbon dioxide.

When Mr. Wheeler released us for a break, news came that our block exam results were posted. Everyone crowded around the score sheet like a rugby scrum and discovered to our delight that we'd all passed, even Tilo and Jones, both of whom had failed multiple quizzes already. While I was still in the middle of the class scorewise, my grades were steadily improving.

"Forty-one students in!" Miller announced.

"Forty-one students out!" added Fowler, nodding her head.

"The key now is to keep your momentum and not let up on the gas," Mr. Wheeler counseled us as we giddily reconvened in the classroom. Then he continued his lecture on intubation, which, depending on your accuracy, could save your patient's life . . . or prove fatal.

Endotracheal intubation would be one of the most advanced procedures we would perform as paramedics and we spent the following week learning all about it. Intubation could save a patient's life, but it also required a lot of special equipment, and it had its dangers.

"If you think you're in the esophagus, pull the tube. If you know you're in the esophagus, pull the tube. And if you have any doubts whatsoever, pull the tube," Mr. Wheeler said with a seriousness we hadn't yet seen from him. If a paramedic placed an endotracheal tube in the esophagus (which leads to the stomach instead of the lungs) and didn't recognize it, the patient could die. "Never let pride get in the way of good patient care."

Fortunately, there were a number of ways we could confirm correct placement of the ET tube.

"You can see it pass through the vocal cords," said Lewis.

"Or listen over the stomach to confirm there are no gurgling sounds when the person holding the bag-valve mask delivers a breath," added Carter. "And ensure you have good breath sounds over both lungs."

Patel added that an end-tidal carbon dioxide detector, a noninvasive way of measuring exhaled carbon dioxide on intubated patients, would also give us important information about our patient's oxygenation status. "If the reading isn't between 35 and 45mmHg, we'll know our patient could be suffering from respiratory acidosis or alkalosis."

"All good answers," said Mr. Wheeler, taking a seat on the floor next to an airway mannequin. "Airway Adam," consisted of a head and neck, below which was a trachea, running into two inflatable lungs.

Mr. Wheeler opened up a blue intubation kit and, using the whole-part-whole method, introduced us to some of the equipment. We would use a laryngoscope—consisting of a handle and blade— to sweep the tongue to the left and lift up the lower jaw to expose the vocal cords. There were two basic kinds of laryngoscope blades. "The Macintosh blade is curved," Mr. Wheeler explained, holding up an example, "and the Miller blade is straight." The blades accessed different landmarks in the mouth and both had a tiny white light to help locate the vocal cords.

"You always want to test the blade before you use it, to ensure the light on it is white, bright, and tight," Mr. Wheeler added.

Next, he held up an endotracheal tube. It was a clear, narrow tube, about the length of a ruler, and had a small balloon at the end, which we'd inflate to seal off the trachea and prevent the swallowing of food, vomit, or blood. The tube extended beyond the balloon an inch so the oxygen we administered reached the lungs but fluids like blood and vomit stayed out. Along with identifying the correct tube, we would want to test the balloon (or cuff) at the end to verify that it would inflate and that it had no leaks.

Mr. Wheeler demonstrated the skill, effortlessly opening Airway Adam's mouth, showing us the vocal cords, and placing the tube, but it was hard not to notice the perspiration on his forehead. When he finished, the class was silent and more than a few people looked anxious. This was serious stuff. The interventions we'd now perform as paramedics could not only help a patient, but also cause irreparable harm. No one had looked at the exit door when Mr. Givot, the defense attorney, had spoken, but I swore I saw a few people glance at it that afternoon.

Before we left for the day, Mr. Wheeler handed us each a thick stack of stapled pages. "Take a tree and pass it down," he joked. The packet had information and release waivers for our human anatomy lab, which was planned for the following week at the medical center on UCLA's main campus. We were also reminded to take full BSI precautions due to potential exposure to blood, body fluid, sharp bone ends, and bone dust. I'd been so stressed about starting paramedic school off on the right foot, I'd almost forgotten I'd be participating in the full dissection of a human body and handling all the major organs. Or maybe I'd purposely forgotten.

"Dr. Larmon, director of the Center for Prehospital Care, has created a wonderful opportunity for you," Mr. Wheeler said. "Few paramedic programs have the opportunity to participate in a full anatomy lab, but it is an absolute necessity to appreciate the complexity and physiology of the human body."

As Mr. Wheeler described the human anatomy lab, it sounded like a grueling affair. "You'll be on your feet for five hours and you will be hot," he promised us. The lab was ventilated but not cooled, and he told us that the protective gowns we'd be wearing would trap heat. Therefore, it was easy to become dehydrated and develop low blood sugar. "You may want to eat before," Mr. Wheeler advised us. On the other hand . . . "Or you may not."

Patel raised his hand. "Do you have any information about our cadaver?"

"We don't," said Mr. Wheeler, "because, in all likelihood, the cadaver is still alive and walking around L.A. right now."

My stomach turned at this thought, though Carter, used to running a lot of traumas in Compton, waved it off. "We'll be cool," he said.

"You may have stepped in guts before, but this is entirely different," Mr. Wheeler countered. He guaranteed us, "Someone will pass out."

At 3:05 p.m. on Friday, January 28, I held a human heart in my hands. "Have a look at the chambers, ventricles, and lobes," Dr. Atilla Uner, an emergency physician at UCLA, advised me, "and then pass it down to another student."

Due to the large size of our class and the small area surrounding the dissection table, we'd been split up into two groups, one in the morning and one in the afternoon.

I'd signed up for the afternoon slot, so earlier that day, Wilson, O'Brien, Miller, and I had taken advantage of a rare morning off

and gone surfing. It was a bluebird morning, with dolphins swimming past us and pelicans flying in the curve of cresting waves. In
between rides, we'd discussed our classmates, the hulking Tilo and
the soft-spoken Jones. Both had failed more quizzes, and Tilo was
on the verge of being terminated. We'd all seen him bouncing from
one desk to the next at every break, asking other students for help.
"You need to get me through this, man," he'd say. "You need to get
me through."

"I told him, no one can get you through paramedic school but
yourself, man," said Miller.

"We can help, but we can't carry him," added Wilson.

I thought Tilo's main problem lay in his planning. "He needs to
put himself in a position to succeed," I said. "Sleeping in the back
of your truck on an inflatable mattress just isn't the way to get
through medic school."

O'Brien agreed and said he was also worried about Jones. "He
just seems quieter. More withdrawn."

"Well, man, I guess not everyone is meant to be a medic and
that's what this program is meant to suss out," said Miller.

We all agreed to reach out to them to see if we could help and
then grabbed a quick meal at a café in Manhattan Beach, where I
opted for pancakes—bland but filling. An hour later, we were on
the seventh floor of the medical center at UCLA, changing into
scrubs, then pulling yellow isolation gowns on over those scrubs
and surgical shoe covers over our sneakers. I tied a scrub hat and
surgical face mask on Wilson, and he tied mine. Then we squeezed
our hands into exam gloves and walked into the anatomy lab.

Dr. Uner and Mr. Wheeler strolled in with us, also wearing scrubs.
Dr. Attila Uner was a man in his midfifties with a buzz cut who radiated intelligence and spoke with a slight German accent. He had served

as the associate medical director for the UCLA Center for Prehospital Care since 1999 and was also an attending emergency physician who taught at the David Geffen School of Medicine at UCLA.

The scent hit me first—formaldehyde mixed with hand sanitizer— and my breath immediately caused my surgical face mask to fog up. The anatomy lab was full of stainless steel, from the tables and wash sinks to the dissection trays full of scissors, scalpels, surgical knives. Examination lights hung down from the ceiling on long plastic necks, casting bright silver-blue beams. A few computer consoles on wheels were scattered around the lab. And the dead bodies were in red plastic bags on gurneys in the corner.

In the next lab over, through a set of large windows, I could see UCLA medical students hunched over cadavers, picking and prodding, slicing and studying. They would spend the whole semester with their cadaver, learning every bone, tendon, vein, artery, and organ, until they knew that body better than their own.

Our cadaver, a woman, lay on an examining table at the center of the room. Her body was wrapped in a white sheet and her arms lay at her sides. She was so thin it looked as if her skin had been shrink-wrapped over her skeleton. Her hair had been shaved off and she wore an ID tag as an earring in her right lobe.

Our cadaver—which Dr. Uner described as an "anatomical gift"—would remain anonymous. She'd received no money to donate her body to science but, as a token of its appreciation, UCLA would pay for her funeral.

Dr. Uner was flanked by two assistants. Dr. Lee was a petite woman with a kind smile. Dr. Wang was tall and muscular. They'd both been doctors in China before moving to the States.

"The purpose of today's lab is to help you learn surface anatomy, practice a few of your skills, and educate you about the major organs," Dr. Uner said as we gathered around our cadaver.

"If you're feeling faint, just sit down on the floor," he advised us. "Don't try to walk to a chair because you'll likely pass out. Just sit down right where you are."

The lab began with Dr. Uner pointing to parts and planes of the body and asking us to identify them, using medical terminology. Then he opened the sheet from the waist up and we inspected the body to see what medical history we could obtain from a visual inspection. The cadaver had a surgical scar on her right lower quadrant. "She probably had her appendix out," said Dr. Uner. The underside of the cadaver's arms and legs was bluish color. "That is lividity, the settling of blood as it leaks from the vessels," Dr. Uner said. Postmortem lividity would be an important criterion to look for during our field internship, as its appearance would dictate whether or not we started resuscitation on a patient.

We had planned to practice intubation but the body was still so frozen to preserve the cadaver, it was nearly impossible to perform a head-tilt, chin-lift maneuver to open the airway into the desired "sniffing position." So instead, we formed a line around the body and practiced other skills where surface anatomy was particularly important—locating the second intercostal space in the ribs at the midline of the collarbone, where we would insert an IV catheter for a needle decompression to relieve the pressure causing a collapsed lung; inserting an IO (intraosseous infusion) needle into the tibia bone below the knee to infuse fluid and medications if we couldn't obtain IV access on a critical patient; and making a puncture below the Adam's apple to perform a needle cricothyroidotomy if the patient's upper airways (nose and mouth) were obstructed and we needed to ventilate the patient.

After everyone had tried each skill at least once, Dr. Uner turned to a dry erase board, where he drew a diagram of the human brain. Perhaps he was intentionally trying to direct our attention away from the cadaver, because that's when things started to get a little graphic for me. Dr. Lee had just propped up the head on a foam block while

Dr. Wang was busy plugging in a cast saw to an orange extension cord hanging down from the ceiling. Dr. Lee drew a line from ear to ear on the back of the cadaver's shaved head with black marker, then followed the line with a scalpel, making a deep incision.

Meanwhile, at the dry erase board, Dr. Uner lectured about epidural hematoma, a type of brain bleed that occurs when the middle meningeal artery on the side of the head is damaged due to blunt trauma, such as getting hit by a baseball bat, or falling. "There is an immediate loss of consciousness, followed by a lucid interval, and then a person soon deteriorates," he said. Dr. Uner was fascinating to listen to, but it was hard to focus on cerebro-vascular accidents when, a few feet away, Dr. Lee had just dug her fingers into the incision slit and was now peeling the cadaver's face away from the skull, leaving it hanging below the chin. Just then, Dr. Wang powered up the cast saw's circular blade and bore in, following Dr. Lee's line. A cloud of bone dust rose up above the body as the sound of the electric motor and a smell—was it the brain?—permeated the room. I felt very light-headed, and I focused back on Dr. Uner.

"The main symptom of another type of brain bleed, a subarach-noid bleed, is often a sudden headache—sometimes called a thun-derclap headache—that the patient often describes as 'the worst headache of their life,'" he said.

Meanwhile, Dr. Wang was attempting to use a crowbar to pry off the top of the skull but wasn't having any luck. He paused. Readjusted his stance and grip and tried a second time. Sweat dotted his brow. He pushed harder, using the full force of his body. The dura mater, the thick membrane that surrounds the brain, made a slow squishy sound and then, suddenly, the top of the skull popped off, and there was the brain.

The brain was yellowish, about the size of a cantaloupe, and had twisting grooves and striations lining its soft, jellylike surface.

Dr. Wang removed it and set it on a surgical tray, then Dr. Uner used a long surgical knife to cut it apart, pointing out the different lobes, ventricles, and hemispheres. We studied the brain and cranial nerves for a half hour. Fascination quickly replaced my squeamishness as I learned that this relatively tiny organ had over ten trillion synapses and eighty-six billion neurons and sent impulses at a speed of 220 miles per hour.

Next, Dr. Lee made a Y-shaped incision down the chest and abdomen, and Dr. Wang pulled back the skin, which even on such an emaciated woman still had a thin layer of yellow fatty tissue underneath. When he was finished, Dr. Lee took a large pair of surgical scissors and cut the ribs, which snapped like zip-ties. Dr. Wang removed the ribs, revealing the organs underneath. The lungs looked like deflated balloons and had tiny, net-shaped black patterns. "Soot," Dr. Uner said. "She must have been a city dweller."

Dr. Lee made an incision in the pericardial sac, which held the heart, and Dr. Wang cut through the major vessels surrounding it—the aorta, vena cava, and pulmonary arteries and veins. Dr. Uner spoke briefly about the route blood takes through the heart and the importance of pushing hard and fast when performing chest compressions. "When you perform CPR, your hands are the patient's heart," he told us. Dr. Uner also spoke about automaticity, which was the ability of a cardiac cell to initiate an impulse, without an external stimulus, leading to a contraction. "Simply put," he said, "when a part of the heart dies, another part takes over to keep it beating."

Once the heart was free, Dr. Uner rinsed it off in a bowl of water and presented it to us. The heart was about the size of two fists and was cranberry red. He handed the heart to Miller and continued lecturing. Dr. Lee and Dr. Wang kept cutting. Out came the spleen. Out came the liver. Out came the kidneys, pancreas, and intestines.

Miller handed the heart to O'Brien, who inspected it for a few moments, said, "Cool," and then gently offered it to me.

Holding the heart—that hollow muscular organ of life that beats over 2.5 billion times in an average lifetime, moving over one million barrels of blood, enough to fill three supertankers—was the highlight of the day for me. As I stood there, a human heart in my hands, I thought several distinct things: I was reminded again of the sacredness of human life, and how the human body was something worthy of being saved. And I felt that UCLA's medical school was validating the work paramedics did by inviting us students onto their main campus. You could see it in the way the nurses and doctors lit up and said hello to us in the hallways. They didn't consider us mere operators of a red taxi with the word "ambulance" written on the outside, but an important link in the continuum of care that began with a 911 call and ended—hopefully—with the patient walking out of the hospital.

As Miller, O'Brien, Wilson, and I left the medical center that afternoon, I realized we'd met our opponent—death. On many of our calls, death would be running with our patient toward the end zone and our job as paramedics would be doing our best to force a fumble.

Wilson had a different thought. "That was intense," he said as we emerged into the bright sun. "I need a beer."

As the first month of school came to a close, Class 36 settled into paramedic school life at the Walter S. Graf Center. The seating chart was solidified. Our food—peanut butter and jelly, granola bars, and coffee—now filled all the cabinets in the small kitchen. We'd bestowed nicknames upon each other, ended each day of class with an hour of pickup basketball at the small recreation center next to school, and had chosen class officers.

Lewis, not only the class comedian but totally dialed in on his skills and book knowledge, was nominated for every office. But he turned down the opportunity to be president or VP in favor of serving as our morale officer. His job was to keep the spirits of Class 36 up, and he assumed his post immediately.

"I would like to announce the first ever Eugene Nagel Ping-Pong Invitational," he said, naming the tournament after the Miami doctor who'd been instrumental in launching the paramedic profession by training firefighters to start IVs and defibrillate patients in cardiac arrest.

"We'll compete in teams of two with a five-dollar buy-in," he explained, passing around a baseball hat into which we eagerly stuffed wrinkled dollar bills.

The tournament took place the following week and was an enormous hit. Personal paddles were brought into school, and contestants sported headbands and athletic arm sleeves. Epic battles ensued, until ultimately Wilson and a private student named Adams triumphed over Lewis and Miller to take the title.

But one student didn't play.

Just after class began on the morning of January 31, Tilo had stood up from his seat. "I have an announcement to make," he said quietly. "I'm withdrawing from the program."

Although we'd all known that he was struggling, the news still came as a shock.

Tilo explained that withdrawing, instead of being terminated, meant that he could receive a small portion of his tuition back and could reenroll at a future date.

"I'm going to get my life in order and join Class 37," he said, eyes moistening. "But it's been an honor studying with you guys and I wish you the best of luck."

We all immediately rose to our feet to give him a standing ovation. As Tilo collected his things, the rest of the class hustled over to shake his hand and wish him well.

"No shame in that, man," said Miller.

"Stay in touch," added Fowler, offering her e-mail.

Jones, himself on a failing streak, urged Tilo to reenroll with the next class.

"You'll come back stronger," I told him.

As I watched Tilo walk out, I couldn't help but feel that this was the moment when paramedic school really began. Forget about the player introductions, didn't the game really start with the first tackle? If so, here it was—the hit-from-behind kidney shot that rattled the wind from your lungs. "Forty-one students in. Forty-one out," we'd promised one another—that was out the door now. As we made our way back to our chairs, I sensed we were all now acutely aware of our medic student mortality.

On the bright side—a seat had opened up near the front of the class. But now, no one wanted to sit in it and, as Mr. Wheeler began his morning lecture, I saw the same question plastered on everyone's face . . . *Who's next?*

February

First IVs and Pharmacology

At 1:15 p.m. on Thursday, February 3, I sat in the on-deck chair outside scenario room 20 about to be tested on my first skill of paramedic school: intubation. I'd run practices, but this was different.

We'd taken the anatomy and physiology block exam that morning—a hundred tough questions on cells, tissues, organs, organ systems, acid/base balance, and homeostasis. Fortunately, in a three-hour review session the day before, Brian Wheeler had prepared us well. Following the review, we'd been allowed to practice skills in the afternoon, so I'd joined Lewis in scenario room 15 to practice nasal intubation. As I'd watched him perform the skill, checking off the grading sheet as if I were the instructor, I'd noticed that my classmate seemed particularly dialed in and asked for the secret of his success.

"The first thing I do is assemble all my equipment," Lewis said. "I place it out where I can see it and in the order I'm going to use it."

"Isn't that kind of cheating?" I'd asked, laughing.

Lewis shook his head no. "I'm controlling my scene and creating a little workbench for myself," he explained, and then he added that he also made sure the instructor could see the skill and hear him. "It's like you're putting on a little performance, auditioning for the job of paramedic."

Now, I tried to remember that wise advice as I pored over my skills sheet in the hallway that afternoon, especially the critical fail criteria—*failure to take or verbalize infection control precautions, failure to initiate ventilation within thirty seconds, failure to successfully intubate within three attempts, using the teeth as fulcrum* . . .

Carter sat across the hall from me, outside the needle cricothyroidotomy station, and down the hall O'Brien and Wilson waited outside the pediatric intubation and alternate airway station. We nodded to one another and gave a thumbs-up: *Let's do this.*

The rest of the class was waiting in the second large classroom, where our skills coordinator, Justin McCullough, monitored the testing at a podium and tracked results on a computer. When a skills station opened up, he'd announce, for example, "Nasal intubation is open!" and a student would hurry out. All the students staging in the second main classroom pored over their skills sheets, making one last attempt to drill the skills into memory. Except Lewis. He was watching the movie *Gladiator* on his laptop computer, reasoning, "It's like being at the fire station. You're watching a movie, then a call comes in and you go."

I wished I had Lewis's calm demeanor. He raced through the skills with such ease and expertise, I concluded that the comedy routines were only to keep him interested.

Just then, the door to scenario room 20 opened up and Jones walked out. His head was down and he didn't respond when I asked how it went.

The skills instructor peeked her head out. "Next student," she said.

Beth Chapman was a hip, good-looking woman in her late twenties who accented her UCLA instructor polo shirt with gold hoop earrings, jeans and Converse All-Stars. She'd graduated from UCLA and spent a few years working as a paramedic in Phoenix. With her bright smile and friendly demeanor, she was one of my favorite instructors.

"How's your day going?" I asked, entering.

"Great," she said. "And you?"

I told her I wasn't going to lie. "I'm stressed."

Ms. Chapman laughed and said I'd do just fine.

"Mind if I take a moment to assemble my equipment?" I asked, heeding Lewis's advice.

"Please do," she said, taking my grading sheet. As I performed the steps of my skill, she would check the corresponding boxes—or leave them blank—and then tally up the points, note any critical fail criteria, and award me a score.

I quickly assembled the equipment I'd need beside Airway Adam, who'd been placed on a table, and moved all the other equipment—spare ET tubes and laryngoscope blades—to the side.

When I was finished setting up, Ms. Chapman reminded me of the directions for the skill. I'd be tested on adult airway management and intubation, and I would have six minutes. "Any questions?"

"No," I replied.

"Whenever you're ready," she said, sitting back and taking a sip of coffee.

I raised my gloved hands. "Let's do this."

Ms. Chapman hit the timer. "Go!"

"BSI . . . scene safe," I began.

"Your scene is safe," Ms. Chapman said. "And you find your patient isn't breathing."

When I asked her if Airway Adam had suffered any trauma, she shook her head no, so I opened his airway using the head-tilt, chin-lift maneuver. "At this time I'm going to place an oropharyngeal airway to keep his airway open, measuring it first from the corner of the ear to the side of the mouth," I said, inserting the curved plastic device.

"Your patient has no gag reflex and accepts the OPA."

I reached for the bag-valve mask (BVM), to deliver positive pressure ventilation. "And at this time, I am going to create a strong seal over the mouth and give one breath every five to six seconds."

Ms. Chapman checked off some boxes on my score sheet and I continued.

"At this time I am also going to connect the BVM to high-flow oxygen, delivered at 15 liters per minute."

As I connected the tubing on the BVM to the green oxygen bottle, I noticed my hands were shaking from nerves. I also realized I'd been starting every phrase with "At this time," which, at that time, I decided to stop immediately.

Ms. Chapman gave me more of the scenario. "Breath sounds are present and equal bilaterally and medical control has ordered intubation."

"I'm going to ask my assistant to take over ventilation," I said, handing her the BVM, "and preoxygenate my patient for thirty seconds."

When Ms. Chapman asked the reason for preoxygenation, I told her to boost oxygen saturation levels and give Airway Adam a reserve for when I attempted intubation.

"Good," she replied, squeezing the BVM to give a breath.

I grabbed the laryngoscope handle, attached a Macintosh blade, and opened it up. "Checking to make sure my light is white, bright, and tight," I said. Next, I chose an ET tube, attached a small syringe, and tested the balloon on the end—it inflated easily and had no leaks. "And I'm going to assemble any additional equipment such as my suction device, stethoscope, and end-tidal CO_2 detector to monitor the amount of carbon dioxide my patient exhales."

When Ms. Chapman told me Airway Adam's pulse oximetry was at 100 percent, I asked her to remove the OPA and stop bagging. As she did, I began a thirty-second countdown in my head. Not delivering a breath before then was a critical fail criterion. I grabbed the laryngoscope with my left hand and then used my right first two fingers to open Airway Adam's mouth using the scissor technique. Next, I inserted the laryngoscope blade on the right side of the mouth and slid the tongue over to the left. Airway Adam's tongue was big, floppy, and pink. Once the tongue was clear, I lifted up on the lower jaw at a forty-five-degree angle. My hope was to be able to find the vocal cords without using the teeth as a fulcrum, lest it break them. When I crouched down to look for the vocal cords, I saw that I had correctly inserted the blade, and I lifted up the epiglottis, the flap that sits at the base of the tongue and keeps food from going into the trachea.

"Fifteen seconds," Ms. Chapman said.

Summoning more strength, I lifted higher with my blade and the trachea appeared, framed by two white vocal cords. I grabbed the tube, inserted it through the right side of the mouth, and watched it pass through the vocals cords. The moment it did, I quickly set my laryngoscope aside. Inflated the balloon and detached the syringe. Then I directed Ms. Chapman to attach the BVM and deliver a breath.

"No epigastric sounds over the stomach," I said, listening with my stethoscope and holding the ET tube secure. "Now checking lung sounds . . ."

As Ms. Chapman delivered two more breaths, I confirmed I had good, bilateral breath sounds. So I attached the end-tidal CO_2 detector between the bag-valve mask and the ET tube.

"What kind of reading are you looking for?" Ms. Chapman asked.

"Between 35 and 45mmHg," I replied, securing the tube in the mouth with a blue plastic device called a "tube tamer."

"What if the reading is 55mmHg?"

"I'd have my assistant deliver ventilations a little faster to give more oxygen because the CO_2 levels are high."

"Good," Ms. Chapman replied. "Anything else?"

I froze. Was she asking this because I'd forgotten something critical? Or was it her way of letting me know I'd totally aced the skill and could end it anytime?

I quickly scanned Airway Adam, checking the results of my work. "Last thing I'm going to do is dispose of my equipment in an aseptic manner and reassess my patient," I said, tossing my ET tube wrapper and syringe in the trash.

"You finished?" Ms. Chapman asked.

I nodded and she clicked off the timer and smiled. "Congratulations on completing your first skills test of paramedic school."

"Oh, thank God!" I said, wiping sweat from my forehead.

Ms. Chapman said I'd done a great job. "And you didn't appear the least bit stressed."

"Maybe on the outside," I said, "but on the inside I was totally freaking out!"

Ms. Chapman told me the ability to appear calm when all hell is breaking loose was a great trait to have as a paramedic. "You'll use that," she said, handing me back my score sheet, "a lot."

As the day ended, Mr. McCullough informed me that I'd passed all my airway skills on the first attempt and had received an 86 percent on the A & P final. I was ecstatic and, as I left that day, I imagined the broad smile I'd wear in the Class 36 graduation photo that would one day join all the others on the school's wall.

But my celebration was premature. That Monday, I failed my first quiz and all systems shifted back to panic mode.

It was a surprise quiz. It was a surprise quiz on a Monday morning. It was a surprise quiz on a Monday morning on medical math. It was a surprise quiz on a Monday morning on medical math the day after the Super Bowl.

"That's just mean," I said to O'Brien.

"Watch it, man," he joked. "No fighting words."

The quiz covered the kinds of conversions and formulas we'd need to use as paramedics, such as converting kilograms to pounds, milliliters to liters, grams to milligrams, fractions to decimals, and Fahrenheit to Celsius. It wasn't terribly hard stuff, but my brain was still mush from studying for the A & P block and as a former English major now in my midthirties, I frankly hadn't seen a math problem in nearly two decades. But I needed to learn the material— and fast—because it would only increase in complexity. Over the next few days, we'd be asked to calculate the volume of medication necessary to administer a dosage, answering questions like this: *Your patient is combative in the back of the ambulance. Medical control has ordered you to administer 30mg of Haldol. You have 50mg in a 5ml vial. How many milliliters do you give?*

We'd also be challenged to calculate concentrations: *You place 1 gram of a medication into 100ml of fluid. A physician orders 350mg of the medication for a patient. How many mls do you give?* Other questions required that we compute IV drip rates: *You are asked to give 650ml to a patient during the next three hours. Using a macrodrip that delivers 10 drops per ml, what is the rate needed?* Eventually, I knew, these formulas would all culminate in one of the most feared skills in paramedic school—the dopamine drip.

If you've ever been in love, you've likely felt the effects of dopamine—the racing heart, the flushed skin, the sweaty palms. While dopamine, a neurotransmitter, is often called the pleasure chemical, it has no such happy effect on paramedic students. For us, the dopamine drip station—in which you hang a small, 250ml bag of normal saline along with your medication above the primary IV bag—was less heaven and a lot more hell. The twofold goal of "piggyback" infusion was to avoid starting two different IV lines and to have your primary line ready to use in case the patient has an adverse reaction to the medication. This skill required us to convert milligrams to micrograms, calculate the concentration, convert the patient's weight from pounds to kilograms, and then calculate the desired dose and drip rate. Next, we'd have to race over to the mannequin arm to start an IV and hang a bag of normal saline; then withdraw the correct amount of dopamine; inject it into a second, smaller bag of normal saline; label the bag; run the IV at the correct rate; and dispose of all our trash in an aseptic manner . . . in less than six minutes.

We were told to expect a scenario like this one: *You've been ordered to administer a dopamine drip at 8mcg/kg/min. You have a vial containing 400mg of the drug, a 250ml bag of normal saline, and a microdrip administration set that delivers 60 drops per ml. How many drops per minute do you give?* Of all the skills we'd be tested on at paramedic school—intubations, IVs, and running a cardiac arrest—more students failed out because of dopamine drip than for any other skill.

When O'Brien handed me back my quiz, I was distressed to learn I'd gotten a 66 percent. I hadn't just flunked, I'd gone down in flames.

"What happened?" the teen asked.

"Just an off day," I replied.

"This stuff is easy."

"That's because you took it in high school last year!" I said, a little grumpy.

I wasn't used to failing. None of us in Class 36 were. We were all accustomed to excelling in some area—in the classroom, on the field, or in the battlefield—and many had succeeded in all three. "Failure" just wasn't in our repertoire. I tried to focus on some advice Greg Hurley, the skills instructor, had given me after our needle decompression station. "In EMS, you're always in the process of recovering," he'd said. "On a 911 call, the incident has always happened by the time we arrive. But what's really important is how you recover."

How would I recover from this embarrassing quiz performance? Wilson and I had made plans to grab lunch at Woody's Bar-B-Que on Market Street. Sure, their beef-in-a-brisket sandwich filled your monthly cholesterol quota in one sitting, but it was also the best sandwich in Inglewood. I was starving, but Mr. McCullough was holding a med math study session at lunch.

"Sorry, man," I told Wilson. "I need to stay."

He understood. "I'm right there with you."

I attended lunchtime study sessions on med math for the remainder of the week and gradually the formulas began making sense. But my stress level stayed on high alert since med math coincided with the arrival of "pharmacology week." Over the next seven days, we'd be required to learn the trade name, generic name, classification, and mechanism of action for not only the medications within the paramedic scope of practice, but also over a hundred others that our patients might be taking. Medications like morphine and Valium had a nasty habit of synergizing with each other, making $1 + 1 = 3$, and suddenly your patient has just stopped breathing.

Knowing about a wide range of medications—not just those we carried in the ambulance—would help us show up on scene and make smarter, quicker decisions. And, of course, there was always the patient who initially denied having any medical problem at all but then handed you a plastic bag filled with orange prescription bottles when you asked what medications he or she took. By knowing the medications, we could guess a person's medical conditions and vice versa.

Our days during pharm week followed a typical pattern. We started off each morning with a quiz that posed questions like, *You are treating a patient who's been trapped between two vehicles for six hours. What drug will you give?*—and then Heather Davis, the program director, would spend the rest of the morning lecturing on a new class of drugs. Respiratory drugs. Cardiac drugs. Nervous system drugs. Gastrointestinal and genitourinary drugs and obstetrics drugs—we learned them all and, with each installment, our fear of the pharm block exam grew exponentially. Jones was now on academic probation, and a bunch of other students had, like me, also begun to fail quizzes.

Mr. Wheeler discussed medication administration. "All medications are potentially poisonous if given to the wrong patient or in toxic quantities," he said. "Even oxygen." We all knew a lack of oxygen caused cells to break down but Mr. Wheeler told us researchers were now finding that delivering *too much* oxygen to certain patients at critical moments could be equally bad. The reason? Oxygen is highly reactive, and in patients having a stroke or regaining a pulse after cardiac arrest, it could damage DNA and cause the energy system of the cells to fail.

As I heard this, I was reminded that nothing would be easy in paramedic school—not med math equations, not memorizing medications, not even delivering oxygen. And next week we'd be starting IVs on our fellow classmates. With forty paramedic students wielding 18-gauge catheters and starting IVs for the first time, we all had the same prediction . . . there would be blood.

I just didn't realize I'd be the one responsible for it.

After lunch each day during pharm week, Mr. McCullough and our skills instructors would arrive to teach us IV skills and medication administration. We learned how to spray a fine mist of the drug Narcan up a heroin addict's nostril via a nasal atomizer to wake him out of an overdose; how to prep nebulizer breathing treatments of albuterol to help a short-of-breath patient with wheezes; how to spread the skin of the deltoid muscle on the upper arm taut and give an intramuscular injection of epinephrine for a patient with a severe allergic reaction. The dry erase board in scenario room 2 filled up with dopamine drip calculations and the mannequin arm for IV skills grew soggy and heavy with fluid injections.

The mannequin arm could only take us so far, of course, so UCLA planned a day for us to practice IVs on each other. Out came the chux pads; out came blue, elastic tourniquets; out came alcohol prep pads, IV bags, IV tubing and tape, angiocatheters, and camera phones to document it all.

After I'd forgotten to push down on Patel's vein on my first IV attempt, blood ran down his arm in a steady stream, soaking the chux pad in red.

"Help," he joked, "I'm bleeding out."

I struggled to screw on the IV tubing but there was too much blood, so I removed my catheter, applied direct pressure with my gloved hand, and added a 4x4 gauze pad, as my classmates poked fun at me.

"You just turned a medical call into a trauma!" said Lewis.

"Quick, man!" added Miller. "Tie a real tourniquet!"

Carter joked that Patel was now in hypovolemic shock (from a low blood volume) and I should initiate shock treatment—lay him flat, cover him with a warm blanket, administer high-flow oxygen, and transport him rapidly to the trauma center.

"What's wrong with a little bloodletting?" I said, playing along. "It worked in medieval London."

Everyone laughed—except for Jones. He'd turned pale when O'Brien tried to start an IV on him so Ms. Chapman had had him lie flat on the ground so he wouldn't pass out.

"You ready for another attempt?" I asked Patel as I tied the tourniquet and cleansed a vein on his opposite arm.

"Are you?" he replied.

"You bet," I said. "Got my BSI on and my scene is safe . . ."

"Mine isn't," Patel joked.

I grabbed a green 18-gauge catheter and flicked off the plastic cap. Rotated the bevel of the catheter so it faced up, and took aim at Patel's antecubital vein in the crux of his elbow. Ms. Chapman shuffled over to observe.

As I inserted the needle, there was an immediate rush of blood in the clear chamber of my catheter.

"Insert the needle just a touch more so the bevel's all the way in," Ms. Chapman advised, "but not too far or you'll poke through the other side."

When the catheter met the skin, I sealed off the vein immediately above it with my thumb. I withdrew the needle and placed it in the sharps container, then screwed on the IV tubing. Then I removed the tourniquet, connected the IV tubing, and opened it up. Drops of normal saline filled the drip chamber of the tubing, meaning my line was flowing into Patel's vein. Next I secured the IV with tape and then threw all my trash in the bin underneath the table. Success!

"Great job," said Ms. Chapman. "Now try doing it at night in the back of an ambulance going seventy miles an hour on a bumpy road with your patient circling the drain."

Despite the blood loss, everyone in Class 36 successfully started an IV that afternoon. Later, as we played our daily game of Ping-Pong, the mood was light and joyful. But all was not well with everyone at the Walter S. Graf Center. If Tilo's downward spiral had been broadcast widely—we'd all seen his hulking frame bounce from desk to desk seeking help—Jones's exit was a silent implosion. He just slowly started drifting away. He stopped sitting with the rest of us on the outdoor patio at lunch and disappeared during breaks. We all tried talking to him and texting but got no response. I texted him: *Anything we can do to help?* Still no response. And then one day I walked into a scenario room with the rest of our team and he was gone. None of us ever heard from Jones again. And now there were two empty seats.

February

The Best Way Out Is Through

On Thursday before the pharm block exam, we had an "optional" review with our lead lecturer, Brian Wheeler. Of course all the students—thirty-nine of us now—were present. "How can I help you?" Mr. Wheeler asked, taking the podium at nine a.m. and opening a notebook.

Naturally, we had loads of questions. Would we be tested on the drug name, classification, indication, contraindication, mechanism of action, onset, duration of action, adult dose, and pediatric dose for all the medications we'd studied thus far? Or "only" the twenty that were on the National Registry medications list for paramedics?

Miller raised his hand. "What's going to be on the pharm block, sir?" he asked.

"Everything," Mr. Wheeler said with a smirk, closing the notebook. "Any questions?"

That evening, I met up with Carter, Miller, and Wilson at the library at Loyola Marymount University for a study session. Carter's wife was a graduate student at LMU so she'd reserved a small conference room for us. The room had a long wooden table and six chairs, and a dry erase board filled one wall—perfect for med math and pharm review.

"Grange, you're up!" said Wilson. "You arrive to find a stillborn and a new mother hemorrhaging after giving birth. What medication will you administer?"

"Oxytocin," I replied, then turned to Miller. "Your patient is actively seizing from a cocaine overdose. What will you give to stop the seizure?"

Miller said he'd give a sedative. "Midazolam, also called by its trade name, Versed. Slow IV push."

While I'd heard that study groups in business and law schools were notoriously rigid and cliquey, I found the ones at paramedic school refreshingly open and fluid. Whenever you wanted to review a certain skill, you'd just state it out loud—"nasal intubation"—and you'd either be invited into a group already practicing the skill or a few shared sympathizers would form around you to start a group. When you mastered that skill, you were free to move on to another scenario room and join another group. We were IV, intubation, pharmacology, and med math amoebas.

Another benefit I found with the study groups was how in a more private situation, students would often voice concerns that they'd be reluctant to broadcast in a group setting. While few students admitted it in the hallways of the Walter S. Graf Center, we were all worried about field internship. Would the knowledge and skills we were learning in the classroom translate on the street? There was no verifiable way to know and maybe it was this anxiety—above all the others—that was behind the race for a seat at the front of the class and the huddle around the bulletin board when grades were posted.

"I was just a lifeguard before medic school," said Wilson. "I'm worried about internship."

I reminded Wilson that he'd been a lifeguard in Orange County, California, which had some of the busiest beaches in the country. "You're dialed in, man!"

"And that's why we're in school—to learn how to become paramedics," Carter reminded him.

"But I'm not going to lie," I said. "I've heard paramedic preceptors eat you alive during internship, so we need to know this stuff."

Wilson nodded. "I heard your preceptors sit you down on the first day of internship and quiz you on all the medications," he said, "and if you get one thing wrong, they send you home."

"Let's study some more," said Miller, nervous.

Carter glanced over at Miller. "What's another name for the antinausea medication ondansetron?"

"Zofran," he said, before turning to me. "Grange, name three beta-blockers."

"Propranolol. Metoprolol. Atenolol."

We studied for three hours that night—reviewing alkalinizing agents, analgesics, beta-blockers, bronchodilators, calcium channel blockers, narcotics, paralytics, thrombolytics, tranquilizers, vasodilators, and anticoagulants, among many others—until the librarian poked her head in the door and said, "Gentlemen, we're closing up." When we didn't vacate quickly enough, she came back.

"Gentlemen," she said, "I can call security."

We apologized. Packed our books and then filed out in silence.

The following afternoon at 3:15, I found myself sitting in the on-deck chair outside scenario room 2, where a medication vial with 400mg per 5ml and a green cap sat atop a wooden table.

Dopamine.

I'd been reviewing med math equations while in the on-deck chair when Lewis was in scenario room 2. If there was anyone who'd ace the dopamine drip station it was Lewis. We'd already nicknamed him "Good Will Hunting" based upon his mathematical wizardry. In fact, he often finished all the quizzes before I'd even completed coloring in the ovals next to my name. But that afternoon, he wasn't celebrating.

"Screw that guy!" he'd said, storming out.

"You didn't pass?" I asked, shocked.

Lewis told me he'd gotten everything correct—the calculations, the skill—but he'd forgotten to write "dopamine" on the IV bag. "So he failed me!"

"I failed, too," said Fowler, twisting her hair in her hand with worry. "That instructor is a hammer."

Just then, the instructor stuck his head out. "Next victim."

I hadn't seen this skills instructor before. He was a lanky guy in his forties who parted his blond hair on the side and wore thin, metal-framed glasses.

I walked in and handed the Hammer my score sheet. "How's your day going?" I asked with a smile.

The Hammer didn't answer. "Take a moment to set up your equipment and let me know when you're ready."

The pharm block exam had gone well that morning—the endless hours of studying paid off—but my skills felt shaky that day. I kept tripping over my words, which, in turn, messed up the flow of my skills. Other times, I'd fumble part of the skill—such as getting my latex gloves stuck to the roll of tape—which messed up my words. But I needed to be on my toes now.

In scenario room 2, I quickly organized my IV supplies, cut a few strands of tape, and made sure the markers at the dry erase board had enough ink.

"Are you in the top of your class?" the Hammer asked as I prepped.

A strange question. "The middle," I replied. "But I'm hoping to end strong."

"I was at the top of my class," the Hammer said. "The State of California should make your paramedic license a different shade of blue if you're at the top of the class."

So it's going to be like that, I thought to myself.

The Hammer quickly reviewed the directions for the skill, then read me my problem: " 'You have an order to administer a dopamine drip of 7mcg/kg/min. You have on hand a 400mg bottle of dopamine, a 250ml bag of normal saline, and an IV drip set that delivers 60 drops per milliliter. Your patient weighs 220 pounds. How many drops per minute will you deliver?' "

He stuck the score sheet to his clipboard. "Any questions?" he asked.

"No, sir," I replied, grabbing a marker.

The Hammer hit the timer. "You have six minutes."

As my heart raced, I quickly scribbled down key points of the equation on the dry erase board:

Desired dose:	7mcg/kg/min
Dosage on hand:	400mg
Drip set:	60 drops/ml
Time:	1 minute
Weight:	220 pounds
Volume:	250ml

I began by converting the patient's weight from pounds to kilograms by dividing 220 by 2 and subtracting 10 percent = 100. Next, I converted 400mg (the dosage on hand) to micrograms by multiplying 400 by 1,000 to get 400,000mcg.

"Five minutes left," said the Hammer.

Next, I wrote out the IV piggyback formula (volume/dosage on hand x desired dose/time x drops/1ml) and plugged in the numbers (250ml/400,000mcg x 700mcg/1min x 60 drops/ml). From there, I

cancelled out like labels—micrograms in the denominator eliminat-
ing micrograms in the numerator; milliliters erasing milliliters—
before multiplying all the top numbers together and then dividing
by the bottom numbers. I arrived at drip rate of 26 drops per minute.

"Four minutes," he said.

I stepped back to review my math. Was my answer correct? I
was too stressed to know for certain and I needed to start the skills
portion of the test.

"BSI . . . scene safe," I said, racing to the table filled with IV supplies and the mannequin arm. "First thing I'm going to do is confirm
my order for 7mcg/kg/min of dopamine."

"Confirmed," said the Hammer. "And what would you use dopamine for?"

Dopamine was indicated when a patient's blood pressure was
low due to poor cardiac output or low peripheral vascular resistance. "And the first thing I'm going to do is ask my patient if he
or she has any allergies," I said, grabbing the medication bottle.

"No allergies," the Hammer replied. "Three minutes."

I quickly "DICE'd" the dopamine—verifying several character-
istics. "Checking it for the correct dose. Integrity of the solution.
Clarity and expiration date." Next I grabbed an alcohol prep pad
and cleansed the top of a 400mg vial of dopamine, then I inserted
a needle attached to a 5ml syringe and withdrew the medication.

"Two minutes."

Speeding up, I cleansed the injection port of the 250ml bag of
normal saline and injected all the dopamine. Tossed the syringe in
a red sharps bucket below the table. Next, thinking of Lewis, I
grabbed a marker and wrote "dopamine" on the bag and plugged
my 60 drops/ml IV extension set into the bag of normal saline.

"One minute."

I quickly filled the drip chamber—which I'd used to affirm the correct drip rate—and hung the bag above the primary IV line, which was already established and flowing into the mannequin arm.

"Thirty seconds . . ."

I grabbed another alcohol prep pad and cleansed the injection port on the tubing of the primary IV. Then I connected the tubing from the piggyback IV to the connection port on the primary line.

Ten seconds.

"Next I'm going to open up my IV piggyback to the correct flow rate, which is"—I glanced back at the board—"approximately twenty-six drops per minute."

"How many drops per second is that?" the Hammer asked.

"One drop approximately every two seconds," I said opening the piggyback line and getting the correct rate.

"Five seconds," the Hammer said. "Anything else?"

"I'm going to dispose of my equipment in an aseptic manner and—"

"Time!" Hammer said, slamming his hand on the stopwatch.

A number of students would fail the IV piggyback station that day. Fowler and Adams, one of the winners in the Eugene Nagel Ping-Pong Invitational, would fail the skill twice, meaning they had one more chance to pass the skill on another day, or they'd fail out of the program. But had I passed?

The Hammer read over his notes. Tallied up the points and, as if it were a tremendous burden to him, signed the bottom of the page. "You passed," he said, reluctantly. "But it was rocky."

Later that afternoon, Mr. McCullough, our skills coordinator, informed me I'd passed all my IV and medication administration skills and also received a 90 percent on the pharm block. A decent performance, but I was still a little PO'd about the Hammer's "it was rocky" comment. Was it ever *not* rocky when a student performed the dopamine drip station for the first time at paramedic school? But if it was difficult in the classroom, I could only imagine how it'd be in the field when, along with the calculation and setup, you'd also have a critical patient on your hands.

I didn't know it then, but I would soon find out.

On Tuesday, February 22, Sir Isaac Newton visited paramedic school. Not in person, of course, but in theory.

"An object in motion will stay in motion unless acted upon by an outside force," Mr. Wheeler reminded us in his first trauma lecture. "If you arrive at your patient's side without assessing the mechanism of action, meaning the forces involved, and assessing the accident scene—you have failed."

Over the next eight days, we would study trauma theory and kinematics, the motion of objects. We would be tested on hemorrhage control, splinting, spinal immobilization, and vehicle extrication. We'd begin running emergency scenarios as a team, after performing a full trauma assessment, and were reminded of the importance of limiting on-scene time to under ten minutes. We'd then test to be certified in prehospital trauma life support. Needless to say, I saw a tough week ahead.

Trauma is greedy. Unlike medical complaints—which often pick folks of a certain age, weight, or lifestyle—trauma affects people of all ages. Not only is trauma the leading cause of death for people under the age of forty-four, it also accounts for over sixty million injuries a year. Speaking in economics, traumatic injuries cost the country over $406 billion a year.

Since 1983, L.A. County has had the largest organized trauma system in the United States; it currently hosts thirteen Level I and Level II trauma centers. Both types have trauma teams and surgeons available around the clock, but Level 1 centers are generally larger, affiliated with a university, and have residency programs.

Together, these thirteen L.A. County trauma centers serve almost ten million people in eighty-eight cities, handling more than 20,000 major trauma cases annually—over 5,000 people injured in car accidents; 4,000 hurt in falls; 2,900 injured in "auto vs. pedestrian/biker" collisions (as if there was any question who wins those); and 2,300 hit by gunshot. Since its inception, L.A. County's trauma system has treated over 400,000 critically injured patients who required immediate lifesaving surgery due to blood loss from bullet wounds, stabbings, traffic accidents, and assaults.

L.A. County's trauma system is also highly successful in large part because paramedics, working in the field and operating under specific trauma triage criteria, coordinate with the Medical Alert Center to distribute patients among the trauma centers in a timely fashion and without overwhelming any one hospital. Critical patients typically make it to surgery within the golden hour, and the less critical patients are routed to local community hospitals.

Whereas medical calls challenge paramedics to figure out *what* happened—is that shortness of breath caused by a pulmonary embolism, a heart attack, or a fight with the fiancé?—trauma calls demand figuring out *how* an accident happened, and that's where Isaac Newton and physics come in.

"The law of conservation of energy states that energy can't be created or destroyed but only change form," Mr. Wheeler explained. He gave the example of an unrestrained driver who smashes his car into a telephone pole at seventy miles per hour. "There are three collisions with this accident—the collision of the vehicle with the pole, the occupant with the vehicle, and the internal organs inside the body." Since the car was traveling seventy mph, these impacts would all occur at seventy mph, and then there was also the rebound impact of, say, the brain hitting the back side of the cranial vault. The size of the passenger also played a major role. Adults tended to go "up and over" the steering wheel, popping lungs like paper bags as they collided with the steering wheel and splintering the wind-shield with their head. Children tended to travel "down and under" the seats of a vehicle, smashing legs and pelvises in the process, and often ending up in the footwell.

For stabbings, we assessed the length of the knife, which yielded important clues about the "cone of injury" to the organs under-neath. When someone was shot, "cavitation" sent bullets tumbling as they entered the body, tearing flesh with shock waves through the surrounding tissue. A bomb often results in four lethal blast injuries—the pressure from the primary blast, which can rupture hollow organs like the stomach, heart, bladder, and eardrums; flying debris, such as glass or metal objects, which can impale people in the immediate area; the tertiary effects of the blast, which can send victims flying through the air, causing additional injuries when they hit the ground; and, last, hot gas or chemicals, which victims may breathe in, and which can cause systemic injuries, including the swelling shut of the airways.

As paramedics, Mr. Wheeler explained, we'd play a key role on trauma calls, primarily by identifying which patients met critical "load and go" criteria. "These patients don't need the ER, they need the operating room," said Mr. Wheeler. The goal with critical trauma patients—those who had a deficit to one of their ABCs (airway, breathing, and circulation)—would be to treat any imme-diate life threats, then get them off scene and en route to the hos-pital fast. To achieve this, we'd need to perform some of our advanced interventions (like IVs and intubation) en route. And once at the hospital, Mr. Wheeler said, we would also have to be able to fully explain the mechanism of injury to the doctors. "You are the eyes and ears of the ER," he said. "The doctors can't see the acci-dent scene, so it's up to you to paint the picture."

To give us a better sense of the geometry of motion as it related to traumatic injuries, Mr. Wheeler showed us videos on YouTube.

They were all NSFW (not suitable for work)—that is, unless you worked as a paramedic. "Really pay attention to the forces involved that cause the injuries," he advised us.

The first few videos fell into the category of people doing dumb stuff—what EMS professionals often ghoulishly refer to as "job security." There was a woman who tried to launch a watermelon off a giant slingshot, only to have it ricochet and smash her in the face, and the unfortunate man who discovered that the rope swing he'd just rigged on the hill next to his house didn't quite reach the water. Next, we watched a video of two high school boys who misjudged the distance to jump from their roof into their pool. Numerous videos showed bull rides gone bad—often with the announcer saying something like, "Aw heck, that ain't good"—and then there was the motocross biker in the X Games who tried to walk off a major crash, only to discover his legs didn't work so well.

Mr. Wheeler grew serious as he called up the next video. "This shows a condition called *commotio cordis*. It can occur when someone is hit in the chest during a critical point of their heart cycle, resulting in sudden cardiac arrest," he explained. "The victims are often adolescents, especially boys playing sports, because the chest wall is less developed."

The video showed two young boys sparring during a karate tournament. Then one boy—a tall, skinny kid—got hit in the chest. The blow wasn't hard, but it was lethal. The boy stood upright. Stumbled a few steps. Crouched over and collapsed in cardiac arrest. Mr. Wheeler said the boy was in ventricular fibrillation, a deadly heart rhythm. "But if he gets immediate CPR and defibrillation, his chance for survival is very good."

By now, a somber mood had filled the classroom, our shoulders slouching under the heavy weight of responsibility. We watched a few more videos of traffic accidents on bleak Russian highways and people getting mowed down at busy intersections in Southeast

Asia. The videos were tragic, but the last one we watched was the most gruesome.

In the 1980s, after a state treasurer from the Midwest was convicted of accepting bribes, he'd called a press conference and, before a crowded room and a live television audience, put a .357 caliber gun in his mouth and pulled the trigger. As his body slumped and blood poured from his head in a gushing torrent, Mr. Wheeler stopped the video. "Hopefully those videos will give you a better sense of the forces that cause injury," he said.

They did—too well.

The videos were horrific and hard to watch, but they certainly drove home for us the lesson about the forces in a traumatic injury mechanism. None of us enjoyed seeing those grisly scenes, but if we couldn't stomach them on the television, how could we hope to run those calls as paramedics? The last thing anyone wanted to do was freeze up on scene—a condition known in the EMS world as "spinning."

We were all silent as Mr. Wheeler released us for the day.

Three days later, as I hurried toward the black Chevrolet *Mo te Car o*—the car I'd noticed on my first day, and which was still parked at an odd angle in the UCLA paramedic school parking lot—Greg Hurley, the skills instructor, told me the scenario for my trauma assessment practice station: "You're called to a car that has slammed into a telephone pole and, as you approach, you see a man slumped in the driver's seat."

Since Jones had failed out, our team was short a man, so I had to be on my game.

I pulled on my exam gloves. "BSI," I said, hurrying toward the car in the hot afternoon sun, where O'Brien was acting as the patient. His breathing was rapid and shallow and his eyes were closed.

Instead of performing isolated skills like intubation or starting an IV, the arrival of the trauma block meant we would now start running scenarios as a team. We were expected to learn the roles of being both a team leader and a team member. As team leader, we were expected to run every aspect of the call, assigning tasks to our crew and ensuring they were done safely and correctly. The thought of having "more hands on deck" initially sounded good until Mr. McCullough informed us that we could all fail a skill if one of our team members screwed up.

"Is my scene safe?"

Mr. Hurley informed me PD had secured the scene, there were no environmental hazards, and an engine with four firefighters was on scene with me. "This is a high-impact accident," I said, "so I'm going to ask Carter to go hold c-spine on my patient."

"Got it," Carter said, setting the green airway bag down next to the car. He climbed into the backseat and placed his hands on both sides of O'Brien's head, holding it still as a precaution for a spinal injury.

"What's my general impression?" I asked, arriving at O'Brien's side and setting the cardiac monitor on the ground.

"You see a nineteen-year-old male who appears unresponsive," Mr. Hurley told me.

I tapped O'Brien on the shoulder. "Hello, sir," I said. "What's your name?"

O'Brien moaned weakly.

"What happened today? Can you open your eyes for me?"

O'Brien kept moaning. His voice was barely audible. I put a hand on his chin and pulled down gently to open his airway.

"Airway's clear," said Mr. Hurley.

I grabbed the stethoscope from around my shoulders and placed it on his chest. "Listening to lung sounds and assessing rate, rhythm, and quality of breathing," I announced.

Mr. Hurley told me O'Brien's lungs were clear but he had shallow, rapid, and irregular respirations. I turned and told Miller to grab a bag-valve mask and hook it up to high-flow oxygen. "Give one breath every five to six seconds."

"Copy, sir," he said, quickly unzipping the green airway bag.

Next I checked O'Brien's pulse. "Weak and rapid," Mr. Hurley told me. Assessed his skin signs—"pale, cool, and moist"—checked for any life-threatening bleeds—"just a small laceration on his face"—and assessed O'Brien's pupils. "He has a blown pupil on the left."

I deduced that the patient was in shock and had symptoms of a traumatic brain injury. "He's a load and go," I announced. "We need to rapidly extricate him and get him going to the hospital."

As Lewis hurried over with the gurney, Mr. Hurley informed me that the closest hospital was five minutes away but the nearest Level 1 trauma center was fifteen minutes away.

"He needs a trauma center," I replied, quickly checking O'Brien's pulse, motor function, and sensation in all his extremities, "so I'm going to bypass the closest hospital."

Lewis and I placed a plastic cervical collar on O'Brien. Carter was still crouching in the backseat, holding his head stable. Miller stood next to the front door with the BVM in his hand, miming giving one breath every five seconds.

Next, Lewis and I slid a yellow plastic backboard under O'Brien, still in a seated position. Since we were down a man I asked if Mr. Hurley could take over the BVM, and Miller could help us load O'Brien onto the backboard.

"BVM's taken care of," Mr. Hurley replied.

"On the count of three, we're going to move O'Brien into a lying position on the backboard," I said as my team took their places. "One . . . two . . . three!"

As we slowly turned O'Brien to maneuver him on the back-board, Mr. Hurley raised his hand. "Let's just stop right there . . ."

Let's just stop right there—you never wanted to hear that phrase during a skills station. It meant that you'd failed.

We froze, knowing a critical error had been made. What was it? And who'd made it?

"Do you know why I stopped you?" Mr. Hurley asked me.

My heart sank. "No, sir."

Mr. Hurley explained that the reason he'd stopped me was because I hadn't done a rapid physical exam before moving O'Brien onto the backboard. "He had a pelvic fracture," he said. "And because you didn't catch it, he bled out."

I wiped the sweat out of my eyes and the hazy Inglewood air burned my throat. I knew you performed a rapid physical exam before transport. But was it performed before extricating the patient? Or was it done after extrication but before "packaging" the patient on the backboard?

"I thought the rapid physical exam was always done after extri-cation," I said, trying to redeem myself.

"There's no such thing as *always* in EMS," Mr. Hurley replied. "Given the presentation of the patient and the forces involved with the accident, I would've done a quick exam inside the car."

That wasn't my only mistake, however. When Mr. Hurley asked me to give a mock radio report to the ER, I realized that prior to starting the skill, I also hadn't fully assessed the scene. I hadn't asked any bystanders about the event. Had O'Brien been wearing a seat belt? Had there been airbag deployment? Was the windshield broken? Did anyone witness the crash? How fast had he been trav-eling? Did he brake before the collision? Was there steering wheel damage? How many inches had the car dented into the passenger space compartment? Were there any additional occupants in the car? "If you arrive at the patient's side without assessing the forces involved, you have failed," Mr. Wheeler had said.

And I had.

As we switched skills stations, I slunk back toward the Walter S. Graf Center, feeling exhausted, nauseated, and riddled with doubt. Could I get through paramedic school? Would I ever be a good paramedic? Had I made a huge mistake in choosing this career? I couldn't help but wonder if the whole-part-whole method was being applied not only to skills, but also to us students. We'd all arrived at school as confident EMTs, and now the block exams and skills stations were breaking us up into jagged paramedic pieces. Would we ever get put back together and feel whole? Would we find ourselves strongest in the places we were once weak? I hoped so.

I stopped at the bathroom and hovered over a toilet, thinking I was going to vomit. I knew I was caught in the second stage of the stress response: resistance. The initial excitement of the start of paramedic school had worn off and the grim realities of the profession had set in—the sleepless nights, constant tension, and relentless self-doubt. In this second stage of stress, I knew, the body uses its stored energy trying to defend itself against a stressor and "make balance" again. Tensions run high; reactions are often excessive; and it's easy to become sick due to a weakened immune system.

I didn't puke that afternoon. But as I exited the bathroom and walked down the main hallway lined with class pictures, I saw a sign posted in a glass-enclosed bulletin board next to our Class 36 roster: *The best way out is through.*

I had no idea what the phrase meant that afternoon. I was too exhausted after a week of quizzes and brutal skills sessions, but I liked the sound of it and the way it gave me a strange kind of kinetic energy when I mumbled it softly to myself. I decided right then and there to recommit myself. To the program. To my classmates. And, most of all, to myself.

March

Struggling to Stay Afloat

Something was wrong . . . very wrong.

We'd finished the trauma block exam hours before and the school still hadn't posted our scores. While it was standard practice to receive the scores in the late afternoon when we combined both a block exam and our skills tests in one day, we hadn't done that for trauma—we'd tested our skills on Friday and taken the block on Monday morning, and now here it was late Monday afternoon, so where were our scores?

A group of us were standing around the bulletin board, staring at the corkboard where our scores should've been posted.

"Maybe they're still grading," suggested Wilson. He'd failed the pharmacology block exam, which meant his back was now against the wall.

Miller reminded him we used Scantron sheets for tests. "Takes five minutes, man."

"I think more students have failed out," said Carter.

"But the school would still post the scores," I countered.

"They're waiting until the end of the day," Carter said ominously.

Just then, from down the hall, the vintage firehouse bell rang, signaling that break was over.

If our written exam results were anything like the trauma skills test we'd taken on Friday, I suspected Carter was right, and we might be in for a mass casualty incident. My team had gotten off to a rough start when both O'Brien and Carter failed the spinal immobilization station. O'Brien failed because he forgot to check pulse, motor function, and sensation on all four extremities after he'd strapped Lewis to the backboard. Carter failed because Beth Chapman—our tester that afternoon—thought he'd taken too long at the start of his skill to direct me to manually stabilize our victim's head. I'd passed the skill but had strapped the tape so low over O'Brien's forehead when I secured his head to the backboard that I damn near tore off his eyebrows when I removed it.

"I'll pass you," Ms. Chapman had said, "but I don't recommend giving your patients the EMS eyebrow wax."

We all passed our next few skills—splinting, needle decompression, and bleeding control—but I'd failed extrication because the Hammer thought I hadn't pulled the straps tight enough on the Kendrick Extrication Device (K.E.D.), a spinal immobilization vest used to extricate a patient in a seated position, when I'd gone to move Miller out of the Chevrolet *Mo te Car o*. They were all stupid mistakes, a result of our being exhausted, and we'd each easily passed the skills on retake. But none of us had gone confidently into the block exam, which posed questions like this: *Your patient is a 62-year-old male involved in a rollover motor vehicle accident. Assessment reveals he is altered, ventilations 18/min and regular; radial pulse 55 and regular; blood pressure 80/52; and his skin is pink, warm, and dry. Which type of shock do you suspect—septic, cardiogenic, neurogenic, or hypovolemic?*

Following the trauma block exam that morning, we'd plunged

right into learning about the electrical system of the heart and electrocardiography interpretation. The material was fascinating, and Nanci Medina, our clinical and field internship coordinator, was always an inspiring lecturer, but all of us had one hawk eye on the hallway, waiting for the block exam scores to go up. As it turned out, none of us witnessed the moment this happened. All we knew was that the grade sheet was finally posted after class . . . and two more students had failed out.

The scene at the bulletin board that afternoon was a strange mixture of triumph and tragedy. Many of us—including me—loudly celebrated our passing scores. But we were in the midst of rejoicing when Wilson and Adams, the Ping-Pong champ, saw their scores. Wilson recoiled as if punched in the chest, and Adams just dropped his head and hurried out the exit door. We all fell silent. No one had to ask. And what could we say? Wilson turned and walked toward the program director's office in a daze.

Wilson and Adams were gone. It just didn't seem right. They were both big, positive personalities and had been major players in Class 36, in every sense of the word.

The rest of us gathered around Miller's pickup truck for a kind of critical incident stress debriefing to deal with the post-traumatic stress of having unexpectedly lost two classmates.

"I can't believe they're gone," said O'Brien, shaking his head.

"Wilson knew his stuff," I replied. "We studied for six hours at my apartment yesterday."

I knew that Wilson and Adams would both make good paramedics one day, and I knew the very same traits that made them struggle on exams—being action oriented and strong verbal leaders—would help them succeed in the field.

"Maybe the school can give them some leeway," said Fowler, shaking her head.

Carter shook his head no. "You're not going to change city hall."

"But they missed passing by one point!" exclaimed O'Brien.

"They didn't miss it by one point if they scored a 79 percent," said a voice behind us, "they missed it by twenty-one points."

The voice belonged to a cocky student named Crook.

Miller gave him a look. "Too soon, man."

"I'm just calling it like it is," Crook explained. "Don't kill the messenger."

We hung around Miller's truck for another twenty minutes, hoping Wilson and Adams would arrive with good news, but there was no sign of them. We eventually decided they'd probably want their privacy, so we all went home to study ECG rhythms. I texted both Wilson and Adams later: *I hope the school can have leniency. You'll both be great medics. Let me know if u want to grab a beer.*

I never heard from Adams, but Wilson texted me at eleven that night: *I missed it by one point. No flexibility. I'm out.*

Every paramedic has an element of the job that makes them queasy. For some, it's vomit. For others, it's feces. And I know more than a few paramedics who grow faint at the sight of blood, though fortunately, only their own. My kryptonite wasn't a substance but scabies, those microscopic mites that burrow into the skin, are easily transferred, and cause intense itching. Despite wearing a protective gown and gloves, I'm still up all night itching with worry after running one of those calls.

We also all have parts of the job that fill us with excitement. For me, I love listening to breath sounds. Crouched next to the patient with stethoscope buds in my ears, head tilted like a composer's listening to the timbre, the sounds I hear really set the tone of the call.

Wheezes suggest a chronic obstructive pulmonary disease (COPD) exacerbation or asthma attack. Fine, moist "crackles" of fluid in the lower airways point to congestive heart failure. Patients with pneumonia often have rhonchi: thick, mucous "rattling" in the larger airways. And if I hear stridor, a high-pitched "creaking" or "grating," I'd assess my patient for an upper airway obstruction or swelling. But more than lung sounds, I love cardiology, which was why I was thrilled to help patch Patel and Miller up to cardiac monitors and watch them plunge their faces into buckets of ice water.

Cold water triggers the "mammalian diving reflex," causing the heart to slow and peripheral vessels to constrict, shunting blood from the extremities to supply the heart and brain. We wanted to see what the diving reflex did to the ECG rhythm.

"Miller's in sinus bradycardia," I announced as his heart rate dropped below the normal 60 beats per minute.

"Patel just threw a premature ventrical contraction!" exclaimed Carter, noting a wide QRS segment on the monitor that signaled a decrease in oxygenation.

Moments later Miller and Patel lifted their heads, to our wild applause. Lewis snapped pictures, and Mrs. Medina rushed in with a towel to dry them off. The afternoon had the same excitement as our first day practicing IV skills on a real patient, albeit with a lot less blood. The diving reflex was why people who fell into icy water were occasionally able to survive being submerged for more than thirty minutes. "As paramedics, we never determine a hypothermic patient dead until they're warm and dead," cautioned Mrs. Medina.

We'd spent the first three days of cardiology learning all of the ECG morphology—sinus rhythms, atrial rhythms, junctional rhythms, ventricular rhythms, heart blocks, and pulseless electrical activity. The rhythms were categorized by the location on the heart where the electrical impulse originated. To perform an ECG, you placed four electrodes—adhesives with gel centers—on the patient; together these offered different snapshots of the heart's electrical activity. To obtain a more comprehensive picture, you applied additional electrodes on both sides of the sternum and in a semicircle under the left chest and performed a 12-lead ECG.

There were dozens of ECG rhythms and, on a critical patient, they often mixed and morphed in a rapid, unpredictable succession.

A patient having a heart attack (myocardial infarction, or MI) often presented on the 12-lead ECG with elevation of the ST segment of the ECG rhythm. The ST segment represents the period when the heart's ventricles contract, also called depolarization, and usually appears flat on an ECG. But when the heart is ischemic, or lacks oxygen due to an MI, the ST segment often begins to sink. As the MI progresses, ischemia leads to injury (and death) of the heart muscle, and the ST segment begins to rise in an ominous tombstone shape, often called "the widowmaker."

There were four lethal rhythms during a cardiac arrest: ventricular tachycardia, ventricular fibrillation, pulseless electrical activity, and the infamous flatline—asystole.

"In V-tach and V-fib, instead of contracting, the heart is quivering like Jell-O," explained Mrs. Medina.

Pulseless electrical activity (PEA) presents when there is electrical activity within the heart but no muscle contraction, and it often appears as a wide, slow rhythm. "In the PEA, the heart doesn't know it's dead yet," explained Mrs. Medina. "And asystole is when there is no cardiac electrical activity and no contractions of the myocardium."

During an MI, the patient still has a pulse and is breathing, but is likely in moderate to severe distress, as blood flow to the heart reduces to a trickle. "What treatments could we give in the field to someone having an MI?" Mrs. Medina asked.

"High-flow oxygen if the patient's oxygen saturation is below 94 percent," said Patel.

"Aspirin," added Miller, "to bust up the clot blocking one of the coronary arteries that supplies blood to the heart."

I raised my hand. "Nitroglycerin, which widens vessels, would reduce the workload on the heart and help with the chest pain."

Fowler raised her hand. "And we could also consider pain relief with a drug like morphine or fentanyl."

Regardless of the rhythm, every patient in cardiac arrest would receive epinephrine—the drug Mr. Wheeler described as a "sledgehammer to the heart." To treat asystole and PEA, we would give epinephrine and try to find the underlying cause as to why the patient had gone into full arrest—such as blood loss, drug overdose, or diabetic coma. As paramedics, we'd use our cardiac monitors to shock a patient in V-tach and V-fib. A big misconception was that defibrillation *starts* the heart, but we learned it doesn't—the electric shock actually *stops* the heart (like hitting "Ctrl-Alt-Delete" on your computer) in hopes that the heart's natural pacemaker system will kick back in with a pulse. Of course, Hollywood movies always show doctors shocking patients in asystole, but that's only because both the flatline and the concussive shock are visually appealing. In reality, you'd treat asystole with epinephrine and attempt to find the underlying cause—what made the patient go into cardiac arrest in the first place—and you'd only defibrillate if the patient was in the wide ECG rhythm of V-tach or the chaos of V-fib.

To practice analyzing different heart rhythms, we patched each other up to perform 4- and 12-lead ECGs. Out came the school's Lifepak and Zoll cardiac monitors. Off went our shirts, on went the electrodes, and, twenty minutes later, Miller and Patel plunged their faces into large bowls of ice water.

I approached ECG interpretation the same way I did learning to surf. Sure, I could learn all the steps in advance, but true proficiency would only come with spending a lot of time in the water. So I paddled into the P waves, T waves, and QRS segment of an ECG strip with the same enthusiasm I had for surfing a bluebird day in Malibu. I read the cardiology chapters in *Emergency Care in the Streets*, pored over the sample ECG strips Mrs. Medina handed out, and bought an ECG app for my iPhone. Gradually, I became skilled at riding the "waves" of ECG interpretation and could identify rhythms quickly and effectively . . . but I realized I'd only seen *static* ECG strips on the page and my iPhone and I wondered what the *dynamic* ECG of a myocardial infarction looked like.

Late one night, lying in bed with my computer propped up on my knees, I called up YouTube and typed in the words "cardiac arrest ECG." A video quickly popped up. It had a running time of one minute and thirteen seconds and all it showed was the black screen of a cardiac monitor. The ECG rhythm appeared in neon green and you could hear a beep for each heartbeat. As I hit play, I immediately noticed a sinus rhythm at a rate of 70 beats per minute with obvious ST elevation: *beep . . . beep . . . beep . . . beep*. But soon, premature ventricular contractions began appearing—*beep . . . beep,beep . . . beep . . . beep, beep*—and then, suddenly at the twenty-five-second mark, the patient went into V-tach at a rate of 163 beats per minute—*beepbeepbeepbeepbeepbeepbeepbeepbeepbeepbeep*. At the thirty-eight-second mark, the patient deteriorated into the scrawled chaos of V-fib with only the scattered, random beep. The rhythm grew progressively smaller, finer, the beeps less frequent, until the flatline of asystole appeared and everything went silent.

As the video ended, I found myself unexpectedly moved, eyes moist, nose running. Maybe my strong feeling was because, without the chaos of the ER and chest compressions, I was able to focus on the fact that there was a person passing away. The death of a human heart. Or maybe, by watching a cardiac arrest without a name or face, I had unconsciously inserted a family member or friend. But perhaps my concern was more selfish—maybe I was just worried about field internship, where as a paramedic intern, we'd need to run at least one cardiac arrest call. It was the one call that tested all your skills, and your preceptors simply couldn't pass you without seeing how you performed. Would I rise to the occasion? Could I nail the intubation? Or would I start spinning?

I knew that with every passing day and skill I learned, I was moving one step closer to that cardiac arrest call, and that soon we'd meet in a living room, an office, or an alleyway. I set my laptop aside, clicked off my bedroom light, and shut my eyes.

Didn't sleep well.

The next morning, Thursday, March 24, I stood with my team outside scenario room 15 for my cardiac arrest, or "megacode," skills test.

"You ready?" I asked the guys, tightening my grip on the cardiac monitor.

"Are you?" said O'Brien, holding the airway bag.

A good question. Like the dopamine drip, megacode was one of the hardest stations of paramedic school, and my heart was racing.

"Heck yeah, he's ready," said Miller with the first-in bag.

"You're gonna rock this," added Carter, holding the orange tackle box with trauma supplies.

"Do it for Team 3!" added Lewis.

And it was then, standing there sweating and stressed in that hallway, that I realized the best part of paramedic school—your classmates. The ones who follow you in the door, who have your back, demanding your best, and who won't let you falter.

"Let's do this," I said, opening the door to start the test.

As I walked in, I saw Megacode Carl lying on the floor. Carl was a full-body mannequin designed for cardiac arrest skills. You could drop an ET tube into his trachea and start an IV on his arm, and he even had a simulation pad that allowed for ECG interpretation and cardiac defibrillation. That day, he was lying on the ground, shirtless and wearing blue sweatpants.

"BSI. Scene safe," I said, kneeling and tapping Carl's shoulder. "Sir, wake up!"

"No response," said Greg Hurley, the skills instructor, seated at a desk a few feet away with his hand on the ECG control panel.

I placed two fingers in the crux of Carl's neck, checking his carotid pulse.

"No pulse," said Mr. Hurley.

I looked up at Carter. "Start chest compressions at a rate of one hundred per minute."

"On it," he said, dropping to his knees.

I told O'Brien to drop an oropharyngeal airway and get out the bag-valve mask. "Attach it to high-flow oxygen and give two breaths every thirty compressions." I then directed Miller to start an IV and check blood sugar and told Lewis to switch off with Carter on chest compressions when he tired. Next, I grabbed the defibrillation pads and placed them on Carl's upper right chest and left flank.

While the megacode was only my second skills test, the morning had gotten off to a good start during the static cardiology station. There, I'd walked into scenario room 5 (decorated as a living room with a flat-screen TV and couch) and had taken a seat across from Beth Chapman, the other skills instructor, who'd handed me four sheets of paper. Each had an ECG rhythm along with a paragraph with information about the patient's condition. To pass the skill, we had to correctly interpret the rhythm, state our field impression of what was going on, and then verbalize the treatments we'd provide.

Your patient is a 68-year-old female with severe shortness of breath. She is speaking in one-word sentences and has pale, cool, and moist skin. She is unable to tell you her medical his-

tory. She is breathing at a rate of 40/min and you hear fluid in all lung fields. She is alert but not oriented. Her vitals: blood pressure 190/120; pulse 130; respiratory rate 40; pulse oximetry 85%.

"Sounds like left-sided, congestive heart failure," I said.

"What's the rhythm?" asked Ms. Chapman.

"Sinus tachycardia," I replied. "Around 130 beats per minute."

"How are you going to treat it?"

The patient was on the verge of respiratory arrest so I said we needed to be aggressive. "Ventilate with a BVM, one breath every five to six seconds," I said. "Then I'll give nitro to open up her vessels and get going to the hospital. On the way, we could consider the medication Lasix to remove some of the fluid in her lungs and put her on CPAP, continuous positive airway pressure, to help with breathing."

I quickly turned the page to the next rhythm—sinus bradycardia—but the patient had no pulse so I treated for pulseless electrical activity. The next rhythm was normal sinus and the patient had abdominal pain so I did supportive care to the hospital; and I ended with a man who had chest pain and was in atrial fibrillation—where the ECG was "irregularly irregular"—so I followed the chest pain algorithm.

Following completion of that skill, I'd hung out in the second classroom (where Lewis was now watching *Predator* on his laptop) until Justin McCullough, our skills coordinator, had called my name for megacode.

"Two minutes of CPR is up," said Mr. Hurley now, looking at his watch.

By then, Miller and I had established an IV on Megacode Carl and pushed 1mg of epinephrine.

"Stop CPR," I said to Carter as I checked for a pulse and looked at the monitor.

A wild, chaotic rhythm.

"He's in V-fib," I said, hitting the charge button on the monitor. A moment later, the monitor was charged so I told everyone to step away. "I'm clear. You're clear. We're all clear!" I shouted, waving my hands.

As my team backed away, I delivered a shock, then told them to get right back on chest compressions.

"Copy that," said Lewis, switching places with Carter.

"O'Brien, you take the airway," I continued, "and set me up for intubation." I also asked Miller to administer amiodarone, an antidysrhythmic medication that might stabilize the V-fib.

After I'd intubated Megacode Carl, Mr. Hurley informed me that two minutes of CPR was up. Once again, I had the others stop CPR and checked the rhythm. "Normal sinus at a rate of 86," I observed. "Do I have a pulse?"

"No pulse."

"Pulseless electrical activity," I announced. "Start chest compressions and give me another round of epinephrine."

At this point, I stood up and took stock of the scene. We had an IV, the patient was intubated, and Carter was now doing good chest compressions.

"What can you do now?" asked Mr. Hurley.

"Try to get a patient history from family or bystanders and begin looking for an underlying cause," I replied.

"No one on scene knows anything," Mr. Hurley said. "But what was your blood sugar?"

I kicked myself, realizing I'd told Miller to check it, but hadn't asked for the result. Mr. Hurley told me the blood sugar was too low to read.

"Okay, let's give the patient dextrose," I said, handing the blue medication box, containing a large prefilled syringe, to Lewis, who was taking a break from chest compressions.

"Dextrose in!" he said, pretending to push the syringe.

Two more minutes passed and, on my next rhythm check, Mr. Hurley told me my patient had regained his pulse. "Now what?"

"Let's get a set of vitals, initiate transport, and do a 12-lead ECG," I said, feeling as if *I* was verging on a heart attack.

"Good job," said Mr. Hurley, hitting the timer and stopping the skill. "Put away your equipment and set it up for the next student."

As we gathered up all our equipment, I pondered my performance. I should've gotten the blood sugar sooner and could've asked more about the event. How long had the patient been down before we arrived? Had the cardiac arrest been witnessed by anyone? But overall I'd felt good and in the flow. Whole-part-whole. *Maybe everything is beginning to come together.* I suddenly felt excitement.

On our way out, Mr. Hurley told me that my patient had survived and walked out of the hospital five days later. "He's now tossing a baseball with his grandkids."

If you followed every step on the skills sheet, your patients always survived in paramedic school. But would they in the field? Was there a skills sheet on how to tell a woman that you couldn't save the life of her husband, the man she'd married fifty years earlier and with whom she'd raised five kids?

If so, I hoped I'd never have to use it.

We took our cardiology block and advanced cardiac life support (ACLS) certifying test on Monday, and all the time I'd spent "surfing" ECG waves paid off. I scored a 95 percent on the block exam and a 96 percent on the ACLS test to receive my highest grades of the course. I'd also passed all of my cardiology skills on my first attempt. While I wasn't taking my foot off the gas, I'd begun to feel as if things were finally gelling. Since January, I'd been marking up the monstrous syllabus with a yellow highlighter as the days progressed and we were now halfway down the back page. Now when we showed up for a skills scenario, I knew exactly what every piece of equipment in our bags was used for, where to find it, and when to use all the medications. How different from that nerve-wracking first day of skills when we did equipment inventory! But perhaps the biggest sign of the rate at which our program was speeding by came when Mrs. Medina handed out shift bids for our hospital rotations.

"Your ER rotations will be split between two hospitals, one of which will be a trauma center," Mrs. Medina explained. The other hospital would likely specialize in some other services, such as stroke or STEMI (ST-segment elevation myocardial infarction) care. There was no shortage of good options. Compton Fire Department rushed their major traumas to St. Francis Medical Center in Lynwood. Long Beach Fire Department brought their critical patients to Long Beach Memorial Hospital and St. Mary Medical Center. Fire stations from L.A. County Fire Department in Inglewood transported many of their patients to Centinela Hospital Medical Center. Antelope Valley Hospital in Lancaster was far from my apartment in El Segundo but had a large receiving area and treated a lot of patients in high-speed car accidents. Harbor-UCLA Medical Center in Torrance and Ronald Reagan UCLA Medical Center in Westwood—with 553 and 540 beds respectively—were two of the largest, best-rated, and busiest hospitals in L.A. County, and UCLA Medical Center in Santa Monica was rated as one of the top hospitals in the United States by *U.S. News and World Report.* However, Mrs. Medina noted that bigger wasn't always better for clinical rotations.

"At those large hospitals, you might have to fight with the med students for skills like intubations," said Mrs. Medina. "Some of the smaller hospitals are just as busy and they'll let you do more."

Then again, in Los Angeles, California, almost *any* hospital or doctor's office could immediately turn into a "trauma center" at any time of the day, as people routinely walked in with gunshot and stab wounds. In fact, it wasn't uncommon for gang members to race wounded members directly to a hospital themselves and push them out the car door before speeding off again—a mode of transport they referred to as "the homeboy taxi."

Given the number of options, and since I was still new to the area, I approached Mrs. Medina at the break looking for some guidance. "Any suggestions?" I asked.

Surprisingly, she recommended a hospital I hadn't heard of before—California Hospital Medical Center in downtown Los Angeles.

"It's a Level II trauma center a few blocks from the Staples Center and Skid Row," Mrs. Medina told me.

Mrs. Medina said that the doctors at California Hospital often let paramedic interns try intubations and, when they cracked open the chest of a patient in traumatic full arrest, occasionally perform a cardiac massage—a procedure in which you squeezed the heart between your hands to keep it beating.

"You'll see a lot at California Hospital." Mrs. Medina said it in such a way that I wrote it down immediately.

As we turned in our clinical requests and March came to a close, I could theoretically see the end of the didactic tunnel. But when I looked, all I actually saw was two more block exams, lots of high-stress skills scenarios, and a three-hundred-question final exam that I had precisely one opportunity to pass.

April

Classroom Finals

The medical block of paramedic school was like an appetizer platter of anything that could kill you. Dr. Baxter Larmon, director of the UCLA Center for Prehospital Care, started things off with a lecture on nervous system emergencies, specifically strokes, which occur when blood flow to a part of the brain is obstructed.

"Strokes are the fourth leading cause of death in the United States," he explained. "Every year, over 795,000 people have a stroke. Of those, over 130,000 will die from their strokes, and these 'brain attacks' cost the United States an estimated $36.5 billion a year."

Dr. Larmon explained the difference between two types of stroke—an ischemic stroke resulted from the blockage of an artery and a hemorrhagic stroke was caused when an artery ruptures, leaking blood into the brain. As paramedics, we'd assess our patients for a stroke with a few tests. We'd check their facial symmetry by having them smile, arm drift by asking them to extend both arms and hold them still, and slurred speech by having them say a phrase like "you can't teach an old dog new tricks." If a patient showed one of these deficits, as a new finding, generally it meant there was a 70 percent probability he or she had had a stroke and should be transported to the ER immediately. We would also check the patient's blood sugar because the symptoms of low blood sugar could mimic stroke.

"With a heart attack, time is muscle, meaning the death of that muscle," said Dr. Larmon. "With a stroke, time is brain, so we need to find out when the symptoms began and get these patients going to the hospital."

The next day, our lead lecturer, Brian Wheeler, spoke about seizures. "A seizure is caused by a disruption in the electrical communication between neurons," he explained. "The brain can't vomit like the stomach to show distress, so it seizes." As with ECG rhythms, there seemed to be an infinite variety of seizures. Mr. Wheeler advised against judging the severity of a seizure by the amount of movement. Rather, we should look at the number of times a person has seized and how long the seizures lasted. "Seizure deaths are hypoxic deaths because the patient can't breathe adequately," he warned. "The patient goes into respiratory arrest, followed by cardiac arrest, so we really need to be proactive about ventilating these patients."

We spent the remainder of the week studying myriad medical emergencies—asthma attacks, spider bites, scorpion stings, infection-induced septic shock, altitude sickness, heatstroke, hypothermia, and drug overdoses. For someone who'd overdosed on a substance, Mr. Wheeler urged us to get specifics in our patient assessment. "For some people, 'one drink' might mean the whole bottle." We heard of heroin addicts whose arms were so tracked they used the veins in their penises for injections; alcoholics who drank mouthwash and nail polish remover to get their fixes; and teenagers who held "pharm parties" that consisted of throwing all their parents' medications into a large bowl, scooping up a handful, and swallowing them like Skittles.

For patients who overdosed, we needed to inquire about what substance they'd taken, how much, over what time period, and whether it was intentional or not. This naturally led to a conversation about suicide. "Women attempt suicide more often, but men use more lethal means," Mr. Wheeler told us.

The material was interesting, but three months of sleepless nights, daily quizzes, and nonstop exertion had caught up with Class 36, and the final stage of stress had arrived—exhaustion. In this stage, attempts to resist the stressor collapse, and you teeter on breakdown. As I caught myself nodding off, I grabbed my notebook and went to stand in the back of the classroom to avoid falling asleep.

Then Mr. Wheeler paused his lecture to show us a video on YouTube. "The video you are about to see is very disturbing," the voiceover said. "It's called agitated, or excited, delirium and is something law enforcement and paramedics are seeing more and more."

Suddenly we were all awake.

"These patients will be aggressive, delusional, and have super-human strength," the newscaster said. Researchers weren't exactly sure what caused the condition, but thought it likely occurred when someone with a mental illness took a drug like methamphetamine, cocaine, or so-called bath salts, a relatively new form of psycho-active drugs.

In the video, a police officer struggled to control a man in the street. The man was shirtless and disheveled. He was breathing rapidly, his skin was slick with sweat, and he was screaming like a wild animal. Two more officers arrived and attempted to subdue the man, but every time they did he slipped away.

"Relax! We're trying to help you," the officer yelled. "Relax!"

The man struggled himself free once again, stumbled a few more feet, and they tackled him to the ground.

As I watched the video, I noticed how my perspective had changed. Whereas I would've once seen a crazed lunatic, I now saw someone with a medical emergency who needed our help.

"The courts, the inmates in jail, and a higher power will judge this man, but we don't," confirmed Mr. Wheeler. "The paramedic badge means we don't judge."

Now I watched the man medically, thinking of how best to treat him. His shirt was off because he was hyperthermic and his blood was likely at a near boil. He'd need cooling measures in the ambulance. He was probably on methamphetamines or bath salts, and suffering from acute paranoia, hence his resisting the police. He would need reassurances that I was a paramedic, there to help him. Also, I ought to dim the lights and lower the radio volume in the ambulance, to lessen the stimulus. Since the man was experiencing an overdose of adrenaline to his heart, a sedative like Versed or ketamine would calm him. And his rapid, shallow breathing meant that he was likely in metabolic acidosis and trying to blow off the acids in his system. I'd put him on a non-rebreather mask at 15 liters per minute, which, along with delivering oxygen, would also act as a spit shield. And, of course, I would apply soft restraints to all four extremities.

As the video continued, the man fought back with a scary, superhuman energy. More officers arrived and eventually they forced him facedown on his stomach and managed to get him handcuffed. But at the five-minute mark, the man suddenly went unresponsive.

"We reached the stage of unconsciousness," the police officer on the video said, before quickly radioing dispatch. "Send the medics."

"He's in cardiac arrest," said Mr. Wheeler, like a coach reviewing a game tape. "Most likely caused by the massive adrenaline dump to his heart."

The police started chest compressions and ventilated the man with a bag-valve mask, but by the time the medics arrived, it was too late. And when Mr. Wheeler clicked off the video, the class was silent once again. Our time out in the field was getting closer. Just six weeks away now.

It seems the moment you become an EMT or a paramedic is the moment accidents start happening around you. If the accidents are critical, your coworkers start referring to you as a "black cloud." If not, you're a "white cloud." Before becoming an EMT, I couldn't remember ever seeing any accidents, not even a mild fender bender. But from the moment I had my EMT license, I'd since found myself calling 911; holding a man's head in c-spine after a traffic accident; applying oxygen to a woman who'd fainted on an airplane; and, after witnessing a mountain biker fall, scanning him for "DCAP-BTLS"— deformities, contusions, abrasions, punctures, burns, tenderness, lacerations, and swelling. I'd also noticed how friends and family started calling me with their medical complaints. My family had always been healthy and hated going to the hospital, so when they called, I almost didn't even need to hear the nature of the illness. My response was always the same: "You need to go to the doctor." But when I heard my dad complain of a sudden, sharp pain in his abdomen that radiated to his back, I didn't advise him to go to the doctor. "Call 911," I said.

Moments later, the paramedics arrived, knocking loudly on the front door. "Come in," my dad said weakly, holding his stomach.

As the door opened, Carter appeared. "BSI . . . scene safe," he began. "Checking for personal, partner, patient safety, any environmental hazards . . ."

It was "Bring a Friend/Family to Paramedic School Day," and I'd brought my dad to volunteer as a patient for our medical assessment scenarios. The idea was to start us working with real patients of varying ages, medical histories, and vital signs. The Walter S. Graf Center was a hub of activity that day as my classmates brought in grandparents, girlfriends, elementary-school-aged kids, and even a few infants. Every student brought in a volunteer except Fowler, who said, "I have no one," in such a way we didn't ask questions.

Carter's initial assessment of my dad in scenario room 19 wasn't good. He was in severe pain. Had pale, cool skin and shortness of breath.

"Let's get him on oxygen," Carter said. "Non-rebreather mask."

"Got it," I replied, connecting the tubing to the green oxygen bottle and handing my dad the mask.

"What you would rate your pain on a scale of one to ten?" Carter asked.

"A ten," Dad said, acting the part with surprising skill.

After Carter finished his initial assessment, he made his transport decision. "This patient is a load and go," he said. "He's going into shock and has shortness of breath."

"What do you think is causing the pain?" Greg Hurley, the skills instructor, asked.

Carter said he'd ask his pertinent medical history questions en route to the hospital. "With sharp abdominal pain radiating to his back, I'm worried he's having an aortic aneurysm."

The aorta, as the body's main artery, carries oxygen-rich blood from the heart to the rest of the body. An aneurysm meant a section of that vessel was bulging and Carter knew that if it burst, it would likely be fatal.

"What do you want to do now?" Mr. Hurley asked.

"A rapid physical exam," Carter said, palpating the four quadrants of my dad's stomach.

As he did, Mr. Hurley told him he felt a pulsating mass. Carter quickly pulled his hands away. "I'm not going to palpate further because I don't want it to burst," he said. "So at this time, I'm going to load him up and get going to the hospital."

"What do you want to do en route?" Mr. Hurley asked.

"Get two large-bore IVs in case we need to push fluid," Carter said, "patch him up to the monitor, and reassess."

"Will I be okay?" my dad asked.

"Yes, sir," Carter replied. "We'll take good care of you."

It felt strange seeing my dad in severe distress, even only playing the role of a critical patient. It brought to mind scenarios and scenes one hopes never to witness. My only consolation was watching Carter and the rest of my team provide compassion and excellent care as paramedics.

Later, as we ate lunch outside with the rest of Class 36 and other volunteers, I asked my dad his thoughts about the day.

"The thing that most impressed me about the students was how earnest each one was," he said. "They've crammed so much information into their heads in the classrooms and now's the time to make sense of all that information and zero in on a specific set of observations and patient feedback to properly diagnose the issue, then create a treatment plan to stabilize the patient. Each student was zealous in doing this accurately and swiftly. Each was very professional, courteous, and caring. I was very impressed."

UCLA had arranged a BBQ in the parking lot to thank the volunteers, complete with large speakers playing music—and a wickedly clever rap song Lewis wrote about being a paramedic—all of which made quite an impression on my dad. He, and the rest of my family, had always been supportive of my paramedic aspirations but I think coming to visit the school really gave him a new appreciation for the stress and rigorous training involved, along with the wonderful sense of teamwork. "This is terrific," he said, gesturing to the scene. "Students, teachers, and administration staff all happily joined together to share a common profession—comrades with a common purpose."

I passed the medical block exam and my medical patient assessment skills test. For that station, I'd had ten minutes to go through the full flowchart for assessing a critical medical patient. I'd walked into scenario room 5, the living room, to "find" a fifty-eight-year-old male complaining of severe weakness. I said I'd quickly perform "V.O.M.I.T." care—vitals, oxygen, monitor, IV, and transport—and get moving to the hospital. In taking a patient history, I discovered he'd overdosed on propranolol, which I knew from pharm week was a beta-blocker used to treat high blood pressure. This explained his low blood pressure of 86/58, as well as his slow, bradycardiac ECG rhythm on the monitor. When the instructor asked what I wanted to do, the answer came quickly and confidently: "I want to continue with O_2, cardiac monitoring, monitor for seizures, and give glucagon to increase heart rate and contractility . . ."

After nearly four months of feeling lost, I was finally starting to feel balanced—the exhilarating third aspect of the whole-part-whole process when the "continents" of anatomy, physiology, scene management, patient assessment, and paramedic skills all came together, forming a brave, new world.

How did it happen? And when was the moment of transformation? I couldn't say that there had been any one decisive instant; rather, it had been a slow thaw—hours upon hours of studying until at long last everything coalesced. I wasn't the only one, either—there was a confidence among the rest of Class 36 that no one else would fail out, not during the classroom portion of school, at least. We'd all worked hard to arrive here—poring over textbook pages and note cards and repeating skills endlessly—but now it felt as if we could toss aside these study tools to start working with real patients and running calls. Being a paramedic was no longer a skill we'd practice—it was who we were.

The last week of classes was bittersweet. Mrs. Medina told us to start thinking about our class photo. Since our class would soon be spread out all over L.A. during field internship, Mrs. Medina informed us we would take our picture at some point earlier, on a day we were all back in the classroom during our clinical rotations. (Technically, it meant you could make it into the class picture at the Walter S. Graf Center but still fail out of paramedic school during your field internship, which, of course, terrified all of us). She recommended we dress professionally ("class A uniforms for the sponsored folks, and suits for the private students"), but Lewis—ever the jokester—had other ideas:

"Let's dress like one of the classes from the 1970s or '80s and take a throwback picture," he said excitedly during one of our last games of Ping-Pong.

"I'm up for going old-school," said Carter, who arrived every morning with the rap of Ice-T and Eazy-E blasting from his car speakers.

Patel said we should focus on passing didactic before we considered our class picture. "We still have our pediatric block exam and final."

We all agreed and raised our paddles to get back to the game.

"I'm really going to miss this," said Miller, just before serving.

"We can still play Ping-Pong on our call-back days during clinical rotations," O'Brien replied with youthful naïveté.

Miller said he wasn't talking about Ping-Pong. "I'm talking about *this*," he said, gesturing around the room: The study groups. The Ping-Pong games. Lunch on the patio. Huddling around the score sheet following a block exam. The bloodletting on the first day of IV skills. Running cardiac arrest scenarios together. The thumbs-up in the hallway before a skills test. The high fives—or commiserations—afterward.

In the end, "this" was that invisible, never-to-be-repeated spirit that occurred only when you assembled Class 36 together in one room.

Patel agreed. "All through the program you think it sucks," he said, "but at the end you realize it was pretty cool."

"Not me, man," replied Lewis, "I always knew we had something special."

Mr. Wheeler delivered his last lecture to Class 36 on the topic of assessing and treating critical pediatric patients. "With kids, you need to start at death and work backward," he explained. "If you're not two steps ahead, you're eight steps behind."

Mr. Wheeler's suggestion also sounded like wise advice for surviving the next six days of class, during which we'd be tested on emergency childbirth, run a pediatric megacode, take our last block exam, and face the pediatric advanced life support (PALS) certifying test.

The reason we had to be especially proactive with kids, Mr. Wheeler explained, was because they were "great compensators." Some children could lose up to 20 percent of their total blood volume before they showed any signs of shock. "But when they crash, they crash hard," he warned.

Pediatric patients posed unique challenges for paramedics. We didn't run pediatric calls as often as other types and, with anxious parents, the scene was often stressful. The anatomy of children was different, with a larger head in proportion to their bodies and a larger tongue in proportion to their airways. Pediatric patients also had different vital signs than adults, and dosing for their medications was often based on a milligram per kilogram (mg/kg) formula that could be easily miscalculated. "Kids are killed by a misplaced decimal point," said Mr. Wheeler. Lastly, it was not uncommon on a critical call to have the parents basically toss their child to the paramedic like a football and say, "Do something!" The natural reaction is to sprint with the child to the ambulance and race Code 3 to the hospital, but Mr. Wheeler warned against this. "A child's portability can be their undoing," he said. "Don't undertreat and drive fast." And in the sad event that a pediatric patient didn't survive, it was also extra important to show compassion for the parents. "People lose their past when a parent dies," Mr. Wheeler said, "but when a child dies, they lose their future."

There was also the matter of child abuse. Paramedics often had a unique view into kids' home lives that even the Child Protective Services didn't. "When the CPS schedules a home visit, food suddenly appears in the fridge and the crap on the walls gets washed off," Mr. Wheeler said, "but with a 911 call, we often glimpse home life as it really is."

As such, it was important to know the signs of potential child abuse—bruises in multiple stages; cigarette burns on the back or on the palms of the child's hand; or thermal burns on a child's buttocks and genitals from being dipped in scalding bathtub water as a punishment. The parents' reaction was equally important: Had they delayed in calling for help? Were they not letting the child answer questions for him- or herself? Were they showing an exaggerated amount of concern? In those instances, "We don't assume it *is* child abuse, but we assume it *could* be, and need to report it immediately," Mr. Wheeler said, "because the next time might be too late."

The lecture was grim, the pictures displayed on the overhead projector graphic, but the day ended on a high note. "As paramedics, you have the ability to change the outcome," Mr. Wheeler said. "You can walk in and say to yourself, 'This scene doesn't have to end this way.'"

As our final lecture ended, I was filled with a tremendous sense of accomplishment. The moment Mr. Wheeler stopped talking, Lewis jumped to his feet and morphed into Robert De Niro. "Ladies and gentlemen," he said, tilting his head and furrowing his brow for effect, "give it up for Mr. Wheeler's last lecture!"

We all stood and cheered, the applause lasting for five minutes. We'd miss all the staff—Heather Davis, Baxter Larmon, Justin McCullough, and Nanci Medina—along with Michael Gudger, the school registration coordinator, and our skills instructors like Greg Hurley and Beth Chapman—but Brian Wheeler had been our principal lecturer and we'd spent the most time with him. And how could you not be inspired by a teacher who made every lesson hilarious; who would occasionally break down in tears when recounting a past difficult 911 call; and who spent his days off visiting geriatric patients in convalescent homes with his golden retriever, a service dog named Ophelia?

But we weren't done yet.

"Most pregnancies aren't complicated, but when they are, it's a train wreck," Mr. Wheeler had told us. And now here it was— presented as a newborn in severe distress.

For OB skills, we used a female mannequin composed of only an abdomen and pelvis. The skin over the abdomen and in the perineal area was detachable so we could visualize internal maneuvers and fetal position. The full-term baby arrived with palpable fontanel lines (soft spots) on its head and collarbones, as well as an umbilical cord, which was currently wrapped around its neck.

"I'm going to place two gloved fingers under the cord and attempt to slip it over the baby's head," I said.

"The cord won't move," said Ms. Chapman, seated nearby.

"Then I'm going to cut the cord," I replied.

I quickly applied two clamps a few inches apart and cut the cord. Ms. Chapman told me the baby's face was covered in dark green fluid. It was meconium, a sign that the baby had been in distress in the womb. I grabbed the blue bulb syringe. "I'm going to suction the baby, starting with the mouth and moving to the nose."

"Airway's clear," she said.

I continued with the rest of the delivery, guiding the baby up to release his lower shoulder and then tilting him downward to release his top.

"You get the baby out and notice he's lethargic and pale," said Ms. Chapman.

I quickly toweled the baby off, flicked his feet, and rubbed his back to stimulate him.

"He's pale. Pulse 80. No grimace or activity, and weak, shallow respirations," Ms. Chapman said. "And Mom begins delivering the placenta."

I quickly delegated care of Mom to O'Brien and then told Carter to start ventilating the baby with a bag-valve mask attached to high-flow oxygen at a rate of one breath every second.

"You ventilate thirty seconds and notice the baby's pulse is now 56," said Ms. Chapman.

"Then I'm going to start CPR," I announced, using my first two fingers to deliver three quick compressions. "Give me a breath," I said to Carter. "We'll continue at a rate of three to one."

Ms. Chapman said the baby's skin signs had started to "pink up" and he now had a forceful cry. "But now Mom is hemorrhaging."

I instructed Lewis to place a trauma pad between the manne-quin's legs to stop the bleeding.

"She's still bleeding," said Ms. Chapman.

I handed the baby to Mom and told her to begin breastfeeding, which would help control the hemorrhage by producing a hormone that causes contractions.

"Still bleeding . . ."

"I'm going to start massaging the fundus, which might also help with contractions," I said, kneading the upper abdominal area like dough.

"Still bleeding . . ."

I grabbed the blue medication bag. "Then I'm going to administer oxytocin."

After I pushed the medication, Ms. Chapman told me the bleeding was controlled but now Mom was in shock.

"At this point, I will lay Mom flat, apply high-flow oxygen, put on a blanket to keep her warm, and prepare for rapid transport to the hospital."

"Anything else?" Ms. Chapman asked.

I quickly went through the emergency childbirth flowchart in my head. "That's it," I said, wiping away the sweat that had formed on my brow.

I looked over at Carter, Miller, O'Brien, and Lewis. They nodded. I'd done well.

Ms. Chapman hit the timer and scribbled a few notes on my testing sheet. "Good job," she said. "Dad meets them at the hospital. They spend two nights there and are discharged to live happily ever after."

Happily ever after, I thought, driving home from school that day. Again, I contemplated how if you followed all the skill steps in paramedic school, your patients always survived.

But I knew the real world held no such assurances.

The day after our pediatric block, we had a three-hour course review with Mr. Wheeler. Just before lunch, Mrs. Medina arrived with our clinical assignments. "Grange, you'll be at California Hospital," she said, "and complete five shifts at Providence Saint Joseph Medical Center in Burbank."

I hadn't heard of St. Joseph's, but Mrs. Medina informed me it was a STEMI and stroke receiving center and that its ER was busy. In addition, I'd complete both my labor and delivery ward and my operating room rotations at UCLA Medical Center in Santa Monica, and I'd spend a day in the pediatric and neonatal intensive care units at Long Beach Memorial.

I couldn't focus on clinical rotations until after I got through my final exam, though. Based upon all the notebooks and digital recorders out, you'd have thought it was the first day of class. The stress level was a ten out of ten. Since any of us could still be terminated from the program if we didn't score above 80 percent on the final, none of our prior achievements mattered much. But I wondered if something else was behind the anxiety: we'd all soon be leaving behind the safety of the classroom portion of paramedic school, and venturing into L.A.'s busiest emergency rooms and trauma centers. Unknown territory. We'd be without our classmates for the most part, working with new doctors, new nurses, and real patients who could just as easily die as live. Gone was Airway Adam with his easy-to-intubate trachea. Gone was the mannequin arm with the ropy veins and thousand track marks showing you where exactly to stick your catheter. Now we'd be asked to start IVs on critical patients whose lives hung in a delicate balance.

Our final exam would cover thirty chapters of *Emergency Care in the Streets*, twenty-two chapters in our anatomy and physiology book, all the online assignments, and any of the material in the block exams or the eight-hundred-plus quiz questions that had crossed our desks. I wasn't even sure how to begin to study. "Divide and conquer," said Lewis. "We took seven block exams. There are seven teams in Class 36. Each team makes a study guide for one block and shares it with all the others." We immediately agreed and handed out assignments.

We spent the afternoon practicing all our skills—inserting tubes into the airway, performing trauma assessments, and running megacodes—until Michael Gudger, the school's registration coordinator, informed us he was closing the school for the evening. I stayed up much of the night poring over skills sheets, and then, at 9:12 a.m. on Thursday, April 28, I walked into my first station for my final skills testing of paramedic school.

SCENARIO ROOM 12—INTRAVENOUS THERAPY AND MEDICATION ADMINISTRATION

I inserted the catheter into a vein on the forearm. "When I see a flashback of blood, I'm going to occlude, or push down, on the vein above the catheter and withdraw the needle and place it in the sharps container . . ."

SCENARIO ROOM 20—ADULT ENDOTRACHEAL INTUBATION

I inserted my laryngoscope blade and swept the tongue to the right. Elevated the lower jaw and inserted the tube, watching it pass between the vocal cords. "Next, I'm going to inflate the cuff, remove the syringe, and ask my assistant to attach the BVM and start ventilating the patient." I threw on my stethoscope to listen to lung sounds. "Nothing in the stomach and good, bilateral lung sounds . . ."

SCENARIO ROOM 1—STATIC PHARMACOLOGY

Ms. Chapman sat across the table from me. "Tell me about Naloxone."

"Naloxone, or Narcan, is a narcotic antagonist that reverses the respiratory depression of an overdose," I began. "The adult dose in L.A. County is 0.8mg to 2mg, given IV, intramuscularly, or intranasally. There are no contraindications and side effects might include the patient becoming combative . . ."

SCENARIO ROOM 5—TRAUMA ASSESSMENT

In my primary assessment, I noticed my patient had all the symptoms of a tension pneumothorax caused by a collapsed lung— shortness of breath, absent lung sounds, bad skin signs, and low blood pressure—"At this time, I'd like to perform a needle decompression with a 14-gauge angiocatheter in the second intercostal space, midclavicular line . . ."

SCENARIO ROOM 2—STATIC CARDIOLOGY

I gazed down at the ECG rhythm strip in my hand. The rhythm was regular, the heart rate very rapid at 180, and the QRS segment was narrow. "Supraventricular tachycardia," I said, "and my patient is symptomatic because he feels dizzy so I'm going to attempt to slow the rhythm by administering the medication adenosine, followed by a rapid 10cc saline flush . . ."

SCENARIO ROOM 6—BLEEDING CONTROL AND SPLINTING

I tied the last knot on the triangle bandage to make a "sling and swath" and immobilize O'Brien's arm and shoulder. "I've secured the joint above and below the injury site so now I'd like to recheck the patient's pulse, motor function, and sensation on injured extremity . . ."

SCENARIO ROOM 15—ADULT MEGACODE

"BSI . . . scene safe," I began, as Mr. Hurley clicked the timer. When he told me I'd responded to a twenty-year-old male who had overdosed in an alleyway, I quickly performed my initial assessment.

"He's not breathing and there's no pulse," said Mr. Hurley.

By then, it was four in the afternoon and I was on my last station, about to be finished with paramedic school skills tests forever.

"At this time, I'll direct my assistant to start compressions," I said, grabbing a paddle with the word "CPR" written on it and placing it on the chest. That day, we were testing megacode as individuals, so many of the treatments would be verbalized. After chest compressions had been initiated, I quickly moved on to other treatments—attaching the defibrillation pads, starting an IV, obtaining a blood sugar count, administering epinephrine, and intubating the patient. After two minutes, I stopped CPR to check the pulse and ECG rhythm. He was in V-tach, so I charged the monitor and defibrillated.

"Continuing CPR," I said, "and I'm going to give amiodarone in hopes of stabilizing the rhythm."

"Okay, two minutes of CPR is up and you find this on the monitor," said Mr. Hurley.

"V-tach again," I announced. "Does my patient have a pulse?"

"He has a pulse."

I hadn't expected that. "And what's his mental status?"

"Still unconscious."

"Then I'd like to synchronized-cardiovert him," I replied.

Like defibrillation, cardioversion uses electricity to convert an unstable ECG rhythm, albeit at a specific point in the cardiac cycle. I pressed the "sync" button, confirmed that the monitor had "captured" the top of the R wave, as evident by tiny pacer spikes, and delivered a shock.

"Cardioverting doesn't work and he's still unconscious," Mr. Hurley told me.

"I'm going to attempt cardioversion again," I said, confidently charging the monitor and delivering another shock.

Mr. Hurley hit the timer. "Let's just stop there."

"What do you mean?" I asked, standing.

"You didn't hit the sync button the second time you cardio-verted," Mr. Hurley explained. By neglecting to do this, I might have delivered a shock at a different point in the cardiac cycle, such as the downslope of the T wave, which could cause the patient to go into sudden V-fib. "I'm sorry, but I can't pass you."

At the end of the day, Mr. McCullough informed me I'd passed all my skills except megacode, but, because of the late hour and Friday's written exam, I'd need to retest on Monday before Mrs. Medina's "Intro to Clinicals" lecture. While I wasn't the only student who had failed a skill—and mine was an easy fix, just remembering to press the sync button—I still felt awful. "What matters is how you recover," Mr. Hurley had said earlier in the semester. With that advice in mind, I drove straight home, sat my butt down at my desk, and began studying for the final written exam still to come the next day.

At eight a.m. the next day, we were all seated in the main classroom with the final exam before us. The exam booklet was thick and weighty and took one of those heavy-duty staples to hold it together.

As for the material, it was as if Ms. Davis and Mr. Wheeler had put all eight hundred quiz questions into a gigantic baseball hat, shaken it up, and chosen the first three hundred they picked. You'd have a question from A & P (*A fracture on what part of the bone may affect the growth of a child?*) next to a question from medical terminology (*Define dysuria*), followed by a question from phar-macology (*What is the dose of atropine for a patient feeling dizzy with a slow pulse?*) and then something from cardiology (*What ECG rhythm would you expect to find in someone suffering from hypothermia?*). On some questions, I was surprised to find all four of the multiple-choice answers correct: *Your patient has fallen off*

a 30-foot bridge and is unconscious with gurgling respirations at
a rate of 4/min. What do you do first? (a) Suction his airway, (b)
Ventilate him with a bag-valve mask, (c) Direct your partner to
hold c-spine, or (d) Initiate rapid transport to trauma center. On
those, I simply went back to the patient assessment flowchart. We'd
make a decision to hold spinal immobilization in our scene size-up,
which came before our initial hands-on assessment, so the correct
answer was *(c) Direct your partner to hold c-spine.* The final exam
was brutal but our daily quizzes, block exams, and review sessions
had prepared us well.

After the final, we all went to a bar on the boardwalk in Venice
Beach for a beer, either to celebrate or to forget. At 2:35 p.m. Mr.
Wheeler e-mailed our final exam results, and we all crowded around
Carter as we waited for the e-mail to open up on his phone.

"Hurry up, man," urged Miller.

"The suspense is killing me," said O'Brien.

"Hold on," said Carter, "almost there . . ." As he opened up
the file from Mr. Wheeler, he smiled broadly. *"We all passed!"*

Lewis raised his glass of beer. "To Class 36!" he said.

"Cheers!" we all hollered.

Miller called the waitress over. "Ma'am, another round, please!"

I'd scored a 90 percent on the final, which brought me to a 93
percent overall for the classroom portion of paramedic school. I
was pleased, but did that put me in the race for valedictorian? Not
even close. I was ranked twenty-second out of thirty-five students,
which frankly, I thought, really showed the determination and
intelligence of my classmates. I'd initially assumed that those who
began at the top of the class would wear themselves out—not pac-
ing themselves for the duration of the race—but they never let up,
staying strong and steady.

After the good news, we committed to our pub crawl with the
same intensity with which we'd thrown ourselves into the classroom

portion of paramedic school. That afternoon, we bounced from place to place, from beachside drinking haunts in Venice to Irish bars on Main Street, Santa Monica. The hours flew by. The sun set and the moon rose, and by one a.m. we were all exhausted. I caught a cab back to my apartment in El Segundo and, when I crawled into bed, fell into a deep, contented sleep.

But I awoke at four in the morning, sweating and feeling nauseated. I still needed to pass my megacode retake. And even assuming I did, I'd realized, the toughest parts of paramedic school were only about to begin.

Two | *Clinical Rotations*

One must not lose recognition of the fact that it is a privilege, and not a right, to treat someone who is perhaps experiencing one of the worst moments in their lives.

—*Dr. Rob Puls*

People will forget what you did. But, people will not forget how you made them feel.

—*Maya Angelou*

May

The Eyes and Ears of the ER

I hadn't even set my backpack down in the break room at California Hospital for my first clinical shift before the nurse was on me. Jayden was a tall man in blue scrubs, built like a bouncer, and had a sleeve of tattoos on both arms. "You're a paramedic intern, right?" he asked.

"Yes, sir."

"Good," he said, slapping an IV start kit in my hand. "I need you to get an IV on a patient, bed four in the psych ward," he said, hurrying to the door. "It's down the hall. And be careful. He's HIV positive."

On Monday afternoon, Nanci Medina had told us what to expect during our clinical rotations.

"You will be on your feet for twelve hours and they *will* hurt," she said, before adding that we were also practically guaranteed to get sick. "You've been in the safe confines of the classroom for the last four months but now you'll be stepping into a petri dish with every airborne, bloodborne, and infectious disease imaginable."

Our dress code would also change. Instead of wearing long pants and collared shirts, we'd now sport navy blue scrubs with the words "UCLA Daniel Freeman Paramedic Education" emblazoned in gold lettering above the left chest pocket.

After the trauma of having lost yet another classmate just that morning—I'd passed my megacode retest easily, but Fowler had failed her dopamine drip skills station for the third and final time—failure was on all of our minds. Was it possible to fail out during clinical rotations? It was rare, Mrs. Medina said, but you could still make a serious error that could break the paramedic pledge of "Do no harm."

The first thing Mrs. Medina suggested we do after checking in with the charge nurse during our clinical shifts was to take a "hot lap" around the ER. "Walk around and see who's in the zoo," she advised us, "and start developing the skill of being able to look at someone and decide immediately if they are critical or not." Following our hot lap, she advised us to introduce ourselves to the nurses and doctors and jump in on procedures—IVs, blood draws, 12-lead ECGs, injections, nebulizer treatments, intubations, chest compressions, and, if given the chance, cardiac massage. With every patient contact, we would perform an assessment—checking the patient's ABCs, determining the person's chief complaint, obtaining a patient history, checking vital signs, and asking any related pertinent questions. All of our skills and assessments would be documented and signed off on by the nursing staff. "If you don't document it," Mrs. Medina said, "you didn't do it."

Along with our ER, labor and delivery, and operating room rotations, and a day in the pediatric and neonatal intensive care units, Mrs. Medina informed us that we'd have another block exam—on the scope of practice and medications available for paramedics in

Los Angeles. On top of that, since Dr. Baxter Larmon, director of the Center for Prehospital Care, and the rest of the instructors at UCLA believed research was an essential part of medicine, we would also be required to write a five-page term paper on a subject related to prehospital care and give a "Grand Rounds" presentation to the class about a unique medical patient we'd encountered in the ER. "You must be knowledgeable, have a good command of your material for your Grand Rounds," Mrs. Medina advised, "be able to field questions and engage in dialogue with your peers, and represent yourself and the school with a professional demeanor."

Lastly, we would need to memorize all of the L.A. County paramedic protocols. "It's time to take that Bible off your nightstand and replace it with paramedic policies," Mrs. Medina said, handing out thick blue binders.

"Man, I'm feeling kinda stressed," Miller said, passing me a binder.

"Me, too," I replied, feeling my jaw and shoulders tense.

Deep down, I think we'd all assumed the clinical portion of paramedic school would be relatively easy—show up at the hospital, start a few IVs, drop an ET tube or two, and go home to catch the end of the Lakers–Celtics game.

Mrs. Medina squashed that ridiculous idea. "Everyone knows paramedic school goes from hard to harder to hardest."

It wasn't that I'd honestly thought life in the ER would be easy. My first experience working in an ER had concluded with a patient stealing my car. I was living in Park City, Utah, at the time and had spent ten hours shadowing my friend, an ER doctor, at University of Utah Hospital in Salt Lake City. At the end of the day, I found my backpack in the triage area of the ER, but not my car keys. Figuring I'd locked them in my car, I went out to the parking garage, whereupon I found my car was missing, too. The thief had used my electronic key to locate, and open, the vehicle. The police later found my car fifty miles outside of Salt Lake City, but the transmission was broken and my camping gear was missing. "That's life in the ER," my doctor friend said. "Some patients thank you for your help . . . and others steal your car."

My first week, I visited California and St. Joseph's for a quick hospital orientation. The hospitals were as different as two facilities could be and still share the same designation. Located just north of Los Angeles, St. Joseph's was the second largest hospital in the San Fernando and Santa Clarita valleys. The hospital had been founded in 1943 by the Sisters of Providence and sat in the glittered shadow of movie studios and the Walt Disney Company. "St. Joe's" was a sparkling, state-of-the-art facility. Patients in the ER enjoyed tasty cuisine and movies on retractable flat-screen TVs, and paramedics were thanked for bringing in patients and treated to granola bars, potato chips, and a small refrigerator full of bottled water and soda.

California Hospital, on the other hand, was squeezed into the middle of downtown Los Angeles. As the only full-service ER in the downtown area, California Hospital treated eighty-five thousand patients a year. If there was a Lakers game or a rock concert, the neighborhood was lively even at night, with parking attendants waving flashlights and a parade of people hurrying to the Staples Center. Most nights, however, the small shops selling clothes and trinkets barricaded themselves behind steel doors, and the neighborhood felt abandoned. A walk-through metal detector greeted you as you entered California Hospital, and the windowless waiting room, with its drab beige paint and strange stains on the floor, resembled the inside of a microwave. Despite the differences in appearance, however, both emergency rooms shared one similarity—they were slammed.

My ER rotations would begin with six shifts at California, fol-

lowed by five at St. Joe's. On May 7, I found myself walking toward
the psych ward at California, about to start my first IV. As I passed
a string of patients seated in folding chairs in the hallway and
strung up to IV lines, I cursed my luck. *A psych patient with HIV.
Really?* As I recalled the blood gushing from Patel's arm on the
first day of IV skills, perspiration dotted my forehead.

I tracked Jayden to the nurses' desk, where he was drawing up
some Ativan to calm an agitated patient.

"Bed four, right?" I said. "What's the patient here for?"

"The usual," Jayden said, tapping the syringe to expel the air.
"Schizophrenic. Hearing voices. Telling him to hurt himself. But
he's been cool with us."

Jayden hurried off, leaving me alone with my IV start kit. As I
stood there, I thought back on the sign hanging in the hallway at
the Walter S. Graf Center: *The best way out is through.* Over the
last few months, the phrase had become my personal mantra and
taken on a physical meaning for me. I knew the only way I would
graduate from paramedic school would be to walk through the
rooms that challenged me—the main classroom during didactic;
ER rooms during my clinical shifts; and people's homes during my
field internship.

But right then I was more concerned with not getting blood on
my hands.

The psych ward at California Hospital comprised six beds, and
the psych patients wore dark green gowns instead of the traditional
gray. I wondered if the color helped security and hospital staff
locate them if those patients attempted escape—or if it made calling a Code Green (combative patient) over the intercom that much
easier to remember.

Down the hall I walked, past bed 1, where a man sat upright,
laughing with a Cheshire cat grin; bed 2, where a woman with
long talons for toenails lay sleeping on her side; and bed 3, where

a woman with unruly gray hair was, at once, pleading and under-mining her case: "I don't need to be on a 5150 psychiatric hold, I'm not crazy," she whined. "This whole city is full of spies and I've been under constant surveillance. People are following me, but I have a lawyer and I am going to sue the City of Los Angeles . . ."

As I made my way down the hall, I grew increasingly anxious about my IV, imagining fantastical scenes right out of horror movies—blood spurting from the patient's arm like a sprinkler, or him grabbing my needle and stabbing me repeatedly in the neck. But when I saw my patient, I felt ashamed for making him into a monster.

He was a malnourished man in his midforties with sad eyes.

"Hello, sir," I said, introducing myself. "I'm going to start an IV if you don't mind."

He just stared straight ahead with a blank look.

"What's your name?"

"Gabriel," he replied softly.

"How old are you?" I asked.

His eyes darted up to meet my face. "Forty-five."

I smiled. "Can you tell me where you are right now?"

"California Hospital."

When I asked what had brought him in today, he said he'd been hearing voices.

"You're hearing voices," I repeated, using one of the interview tactics I'd learned. "Please go on."

Gabriel said he'd been hearing voices the night before, but wasn't hearing them anymore now.

"That's good," I said, quickly checking his ABCs and finding no deficits. When I checked his radial pulse, I noticed his veins were supercharged and ropy, which, in this case, was more worrisome than him having no veins. I would have no issue finding a vein, but what would happen when I did? Again, I imagined a blood geyser spurting everywhere.

With the tourniquet on and site clean, I ensured the bag of IV fluid was normal saline, the correct amount, and not expired. Next, I attached the IV tubing to the bag and ran it open for a moment so all the air bubbles disappeared, lest they enter the patient's circulation and block a vein or artery. Next, I grabbed my 18-gauge catheter and stabilized a vein with my left hand. "You're just going to feel a little pinch," I said, taking aim.

"Do what you gotta do," he replied.

I took a breath. Steadied my aim and inserted the catheter into the vein. "Poke and pray," as they say. Blood filled the green catheter in seconds—more a tiny flood than a flash. I advanced the catheter, then occluded the vein above the injection site with my left thumb and removed the needle, placing it in a red sharps container to the right of the bed. Next I attached the IV tubing and applied a clear securement dressing to hold the IV in place. Then I stood up to assess my work—it was a perfectly placed IV without a drop of spilled blood. Success!

"Have a great day, sir," I said, walking off.

"You, too," he replied.

Following my first IV, I had a moment to introduce myself to everyone. The ER was large and had a nursing station at the center, but I found the doctors and nursing staff scattered around in varying states of stress and activity—patching up a patient to the ECG machine, helping a new arrival change into her gown, punching in the security code on a locked cabinet full of medications, inserting an implanted urinary catheter, and even grabbing a patient some butter for his breakfast roll.

"A paramedic intern? Oh, good!" said a nurse named Aliyah, smiling. "Now we have someone to abuse!"

As I met the other nurses, I discovered many were guys who

had once dreamed of working for the fire department as firefighters and paramedics.

"I sure miss the field," said Mateo, a nurse in his late twenties who had worked as an EMT. "Nothing better than having a great partner and rolling through the streets of L.A. saving lives!"

"How come you switched careers?" I asked.

"I wasn't getting hired," he replied, explaining that, even with firefighter training and his EMT license, there were thousands of other applicants vying for each position.

In Mateo's eyes—and the others I spoke with—I saw a longing for the field that was reminiscent of sailors who'd left the sea to work on the ships in port.

I had tried not to think about job prospects during paramedic school. I'd wanted to focus solely on my studies . . . and maybe I also hadn't wanted to face the odds. Getting hired by a large department like L.A. City or L.A. County was not unlike winning the lottery. But there was a noble reason for Mateo's career change to nursing. "I had mouths to feed and needed a career to support my family."

I told Mateo to grab me if he needed anything and continued my hot lap.

Critical, I thought, seeing a pale man in his fifties who had overdosed on aspirin.

"Hey, how are you?" he said to me, waving me over.

"Fine, thanks," I replied. "Can I get you anything?"

He shook his head no. "I just feel a little sick."

"Want me to get you something for the nausea?" I asked.

Again he shook his head no. "I'll be fine."

But I knew he wouldn't be. Sure, he was sitting up and talking to me—there was no deficit to his ABCs—but Aliyah had told me he'd swallowed far more than the suggested dose, and I knew he would deteriorate. Following this period of malaise, he'd likely feel increasing tenderness in the right upper quadrant of his abdomen and, within seventy-two to ninety-six hours, metabolic acidosis would set in, causing irreparable kidney and liver failure. Sadly, an aspirin overdose was one condition that even a hospital sometimes couldn't fix. I was likely talking to a corpse.

Not critical, I thought, passing a seventy-one-year-old man with flu symptoms and stable vital signs. Ditto a forty-seven-year-old woman complaining of anxiety. I passed two middle-aged men in adjacent beds who'd both come to the ER for chest pain and a woman of similar age who'd had a seizure, with no history of them—*all critical*. As I recalled from didactic, "time is muscle" in cases of a heart attack; and it wasn't normal for someone in middle age to suddenly start having seizures. The next patient was a seventy-five-year-old woman who'd had a headache for three days and presented in no distress. *Not critical*, I thought . . . but I wanted to find out more of her history: Had she suffered any recent trauma? Did she have any vision disturbances? How was her hearing? I wanted to rule out a brain bleed or hypertensive (high blood pressure) crisis.

Following her, I saw a man reeking of alcohol who'd fallen and had an altered level of consciousness. Was he altered from drinking? Or was he not responding appropriately because he'd hit his head and now had a traumatic brain injury? *Critical*, I thought, swaying on the side of safety. The next patient was a twenty-four-year-old female who was two months pregnant with severe abdominal pain. Morning sickness? Or an ectopic pregnancy? *Critical*, I decided.

"Critical" didn't necessarily mean the patients were at death's door. Rather, it just meant that, as a paramedic in the field and based upon their chief complaint, I would have a high index of suspicion and err on the side of safety. Similarly, when I rated someone "not critical," it didn't mean they couldn't become critical at a moment's notice.

I met an elderly couple from Utah in the next room. They'd been driving from Utah to San Diego to see their grandkids when the man started to have chest pain, so they stopped at the first hospital they could find.

"Nice to meet you, Daniel," the man said, reading the name on my scrubs.

"Actually, Daniel Freeman is a paramedic school," I said. "My name is—"

"Wow, a paramedic, Daniel," the man interjected. "God bless you."

When the man introduced himself as Earl, I told him my name was Kevin.

"Well, Daniel, I'd like you to meet my wife, Marilyn," he replied, not hearing me.

"Nice to meet you," I said, resolving myself to my new nickname.

"Been married to this one fifty-two years," Earl said, as I listened to his breath sounds. "Best decision I ever made."

Earl had come in with a chest pain that radiated to his jaw. His ECG showed no sign of heart attack and his cardiac enzyme labs also came back normal, but his cholesterol was elevated and he had a history of high blood pressure, so the hospital wanted to keep him overnight to monitor him. I thanked Earl and Marilyn for their time and continued on.

"'Bye, Daniel," he replied, waving. "Come back and visit, y'hear?"

As I finished my hot lap, Aliyah, Mateo, and the other nurses started giving me jobs. By now, the ER was full and paramedics from LAFD and a number of private ambulance companies were rushing patients in. ECGs, vital signs, blood draws, intramuscular injections, IV injections, blood sugar checks—I did it all—and when paramedics from LAFD brought in a young man who'd been shot that afternoon, I attempted my first IV on a major trauma patient.

"How's the IV?" yelled Mateo, surrounded by a team of doctors and nurses. "He needs fluid!"

"I got it," I said, taking aim at the vein.

Luciano was a twenty-one-year-old guy with a shaved head and goatee. He wore a white T-shirt, with a rosary around his neck, and his baggy jean shorts were soaked with blood. He'd been standing outside when a Toyota Corolla sped by and someone shot him in his upper thigh. His leg looked swollen, so there was a chance the bullet had severed his femoral artery.

I tied off my IV tourniquet and cleansed the top of his hand. Took aim and inserted the catheter. But no blood filled the catheter chamber. I maneuvered the needle around, hoping to find the vein, as Luciano howled in pain. The pain could have been from the gunshot wound . . . or from me fishing around for a vein.

"Take it out and try again," Mateo instructed.

"We need that IV," said the doctor, a tall, blond man.

I withdrew the catheter and set it on the surgical tray next to the bed. Grabbed another catheter, cleansed the site, and tried at another vein on his forearm.

"Where's the IV?" yelled the doctor.

"Coming," I said, searching around with my needle again, hoping for a flashback of blood.

"Ouch!" yelled Luciano. "Man, what are you doing?"

Mateo instructed me to withdraw my needle. "I'll take it from here," he said before effortlessly placing an IV moments later. As I slunk out of the room, I noticed Luciano giving me a hard stare.

Missing Luciano's IV seemed to put me in a slump with every IV for the rest of the shift. It was like the veins all got together and said, "Let's play a game of hide-and-seek with the new guy!" Forget missing an IV—on many patients I couldn't even *find* a vein to make an attempt. Most of the patients off Skid Row were skeletal thin and you could only see tendons popping out of their arms.

Other patients' veins were hidden behind thick layers of fatty tissue. On some patients, I spotted veins lining the surface of their hands or arms, but they were terribly thin and spidery. Other times, I would palpate a suitable vein and tie off my tourniquet, only to have it suddenly disappear when I took aim with my catheter. "Don't let it get to you," one man told me. "My veins run like Emmitt Smith." Other veins rolled when I poked them. And on another patient—a young guy who'd come in with an elevated blood sugar—I immediately saw a flashback when I inserted my catheter, only to have the blood flow suddenly stop moments later.

"You hit a valve," Aliyah said, walking past. "Try again on the other arm."

My inability to get an IV that day felt awful and, again, my worries about field internship returned—how could I pass that, if I couldn't handle something this simple? Like a gambler who continued to bet despite mounting losses, I kept trying IVs for the next five hours, aiming and firing, poking and praying. I became so engrossed in trying to perfect IVs that I forgot to take a lunch break. By nine p.m., I felt sick; my feet ached; and I had a pounding headache. By then, Aliyah and Mateo and the rest of the nurses had left for the day, turning over the care of their patients to a new, caffeinated crop of nurses, many of them fresh out of school themselves.

Exhausted, I decided to grab a granola bar from my backpack, but before I could, a voice called out to me: "Hey, Daniel!"

It was Earl from Utah. His wife was asleep in the chair next to his bed and he looked hungry for company.

"How's it going?" I said, standing at the doorway.

"Wonderful, Mr. Freeman," he replied. "Every day a holiday. Every meal a banquet."

I laughed and said he should get some sleep.

"Sleep is overrated," he replied, waving me in. I looked over at his wife. "Aw, don't worry about her," he said. "Nothing wakes her."

I pondered my options. Technically, I was at California Hospital to practice my skills. Then again, maybe my mantra—*the best way out is through*—didn't apply just to rooms that challenged me, but also to rooms that taught and inspired me.

Like this one.

I walked in and sat down. I ended up spending a half hour with Earl, learning about his childhood and life on the farm. We didn't talk medicine but, for some reason, all my worries about paramedic school and my IV skills disappeared. Some people are like that— they make you feel better just by their smile and the kindness in their eyes.

Earl yawned. "Say, what are you studying to become again, Daniel?"

"A paramedic," I replied.

"How wonderful," he said, and I could tell by the tone in his voice that paramedics had responded to his house for him or his wife in the past. Then he took my hand—as if I'd been the paramedic who'd treated him—and said, "Thank you, son . . . Thank you."

On my next shift at California Hospital, I attempted my first intubation on a real patient. It happened around lunchtime. Aliyah had told me to start an IV on a patient in bed 7. Paramedics had responded near Skid Row—an area that three thousand to six thousand homeless people call home—for a woman having a seizure. The patient, a rail-thin woman in her late forties, wasn't seizing when the paramedics arrived on scene but she was lethargic and altered. One bystander said the woman had had one seizure lasting ten minutes. "No, she had five seizures lasting one minute each," offered another man. A third bystander said the woman had actually died and he'd revived her with his telepathic powers, which prompted the paramedic to tell the guys on the engine, "Let's just c-spine her and get going to California Hospital." So now here she was in bed 7, still lethargic and not answering questions appropriately, with me scrubbing her right forearm with an alcohol prep pad. The woman wore a blue tank top, sweatpants, and plastic grocery bags for shoes. I had to use five alcohol prep pads just to wipe the dirt off her arm. Once the spot was clean, I grabbed an 18-gauge catheter and took aim at the dorsal vein that traveled in the canyon atop her hand, between her fourth finger and pinkie. "You're going to feel a little pinch," I said, focusing on the IV.

The moment the needle pierced her skin, the woman's eyes rolled back in her head and her whole body became rigid. Her arms pulled toward the center of her body and she emitted a moan as air was forcefully expelled through her vocal cords. She was having a tonic-clonic seizure. I quickly withdrew my needle and yelled out to Aliyah, "I need some help in here!"

I grabbed a non-rebreather mask and attached the tubing to the oxygen port on the wall. Cranked it up to 15 liters per minute and positioned it over the woman's mouth, then quickly placed her bed pillows on the rails so she didn't hurt herself. Aliyah arrived with Ativan, a sedative to control the seizure. By now the woman was in the clonic phase, her arms and legs jerking rhythmically. When the seizure activity subsided a moment later, I held the woman's left arm taut as Aliyah quickly got an IV in. But no sooner had we secured the IV than the woman started seizing again.

Aliyah handed me the syringe with Ativan. "Go ahead and administer this," she said. "Adjust your dose to seizure activity." Once I'd given her some of the medication, the woman stopped seizing.

Meanwhile, Dr. Schultz, a small woman with glasses, had arrived. "We need to RSI her—she can't protect her airway."

RSI, or rapid sequence intubation, was a medical procedure that used the prompt induction of a sedative and short-term paralytic to facilitate intubation and control the patient's airway. Initiating unconsciousness and paralysis in the patient made intubation easier, but it was also a high-risk procedure because you were essentially putting the patient in respiratory arrest. Any patient requiring RSI is already critical to begin with. Along with temporarily stopping breathing, RSI also relaxed the lower sphincter muscles on the esophagus, which increased the likelihood of the patient aspirating her stomach contents—precisely the condition we were trying to avoid. And as if that wasn't enough, the introduction of an endotracheal tube could potentially stimulate our patient's vagus nerve, causing her blood pressure to tank, resulting in cardiac arrest. Or, on the flip side, if the doctors hadn't given enough of the sedative medication, the patient's adrenal system may activate, sending her pulse through the roof, which could also cause cardiac arrest.

I asked Dr. Schultz if I could get the intubation.

"You think you're ready?" she asked.

"Yes, ma'am," I replied confidently.

"Okay, then," said Dr. Schultz. "But if you don't see the vocal cords immediately, I want you to hand it off."

"Volunteer any chance you can in paramedic school," my friend Patrick, a physician assistant, had said to me before I started. "You'll be scared shitless when you attempt a procedure for the first time but I guarantee you'll learn a hell of a lot more than those scared students hanging in back." So here I was, preparing to test the balloon cuff on my 7.0mm ET tube and make sure the light on the laryngoscope blade was "white, bright, and tight," with about half the ER watching.

Following Dr. Schultz's orders for an RSI, there was a great rush of activity beside bed 7.

A nurse rolled over the intubation trolley, a blue cabinet on four wheels. Out came a laryngoscope handle and blades of varying size and shape. Out came an oropharyngeal airway and bag-valve mask, along with an assortment of endotracheal tubes, syringes, an end-tidal CO_2 detector, and suction equipment. Nearby, Aliyah drew up the medication etomidate, a short-term anesthetic agent, and succinylcholine, the short-acting paralytic we'd use. When the respiratory therapist arrived, he slipped a pillow under the patient's head to move it into the sniffing position. He dropped the airway into her mouth and began ventilating the patient with the mask to preoxygenate her. Our goal was to wash all the nitrogen out of her system and raise the oxygen saturation in her blood to 100 percent.

"The patient's been preoxygenated for four minutes and is at 100 percent," the respiratory therapist said.

Dr. Schultz turned to Aliyah. "Go ahead and push the etomidate."

"Etomidate going in now," Aliyah replied, following the injection with a 10cc flush of normal saline.

Dr. Schultz waited about twenty seconds and then instructed Aliyah to administer the succinylcholine.

"Succs going in now . . ."

I stood at the head of the bed with the laryngoscope in my left hand, waiting. As the respiratory therapist continued to ventilate, the woman's chest rose and fell peacefully. I checked the pulse oximetry on the monitor: still 100 percent. Just then, the muscles in the patient's neck began twitching. It looked as if bugs were crawling under her skin.

Dr. Schultz said such involuntary muscle twitches were normal during RSI. "They're called *fasciculations* and result from the spontaneous depolarization of the lower motor neurons." A moment later, Dr. Schultz stepped aside and gestured to the head of the bed. "Whenever you're ready."

I asked the respiratory therapist to stop bagging and remove the OPA on the count of three.

"One . . . two . . . three," I said, tightening my grip on the laryngoscope.

The respiratory therapist stepped aside and pushed down on the patient's cricoid cartilage in her neck, a process known as "cric pressure." This would help to reveal the glottic opening and to seal off the esophagus, preventing aspiration of stomach contents. Leaning in close, I used the first two fingers of my right hand to scissor the patient's mouth open and inserted the laryngoscope blade with my left hand. I worked slowly, mindful not to pinch the gums or the teeth.

When I looked in the mouth, I suddenly realized a real patient was nothing like Airway Adam. All I saw was tongue, saliva, and teeth. As I tried to sweep the tongue to the left, it fell off my blade handle to the right. When I tried to corral it again, the slippery slab dropped to the left.

"Twenty seconds," said Aliyah, counting down my remaining time. I had to finish my intubation in less than thirty seconds, or the patient's oxygen levels would drop rapidly.

I gently maneuvered the laryngoscope back to the right and tilted my blade down to scoop the tongue up again. Maintaining that angle, I swept it delicately over to the left and lifted up on the lower jaw.

"Fifteen seconds."

I peered in close, expecting to see the vocal cords. But once again, all I saw was pink gum and white teeth.

"Lift a little higher," instructed Dr. Schultz, leaning in behind me.

I hadn't guessed a patient's head would weigh so much. Summoning all my strength, I lifted it up and leaned in for another look—still nothing.

Aliyah told me I had ten seconds left.

Dr. Schultz peered in over my shoulder. "See anything?"

"Nothing," I replied, lowering the patient's head and removing my blade.

The respiratory therapist quickly rushed in to reoxygenate the patient. When her oxygen level was back up to 100 percent, Dr. Schultz inserted the laryngoscope blade, swept the tongue to the left, and lifted up on the lower jaw.

"Tube, please," she said, opening her hand. "See the vocal cords?"

I leaned in and there they were—framing the opening to the trachea in white.

Aliyah handed her the ET tube and Dr. Schultz effortlessly placed it in the trachea.

"Everyone has trouble the first time," she said, removing her safety gloves and tossing them into the trash. "Keep practicing."

The next day, I was back in the main classroom of the Walter S. Graf Center for Nanci Medina's lecture on L.A. County paramedic protocols. "Policy 814 outlines how paramedics can determine death in the field," she said. "And there are numerous different ways."

The L.A. County paramedic protocols outlined the scope of practice, or treatments, we could provide during our internship. We'd be required to learn all the protocols, but would use some more than others. "Policy 806 outlines what treatments we can provide prior to contacting our base hospital, and Policy 808 outlines when base contact and patient transport are mandatory."

Policies 510 through 513 concerned where we should transport pediatric and pregnant patients, burn victims, and people suffering from heart attacks. The hospital destination was critically important for a patient's survival. For instance, if your patient was having a heart attack, it was better to bypass the closest emergency room and travel ten minutes up the road to a STEMI receiving center.

Policy 506 outlined which patients should be transported to a trauma center.

"Think of it this way," Lewis advised us fellow students, tilting back on his chair to draw in his audience. "If people drive backward on the 605 Freeway in Los Angeles, they're going to need Policy 506 for trauma triage."

Policy 521 concerned stroke patient destination; Policy 815 told us what documentation was acceptable as a do-not-resuscitate order—"and a 'DNR' tattoo on their chest doesn't count," added Mrs. Medina—and Policy 814 concerned when a paramedic should render no treatment, because the patient was dead.

"A person may be determined dead if, in the absence of breathing, a pulse, and neurological reflexes, one or more of these conditions exist," Mrs. Medina said, reading: "Decapitation. Decomposition. Incineration. A massive crush injury. A penetrating or blunt injury with evisceration of the heart, lung, or brain."

With each condition she mentioned, my mind quickly filled in the blanks with horrific images. I felt the fish taco I'd had for lunch swimming laps in my stomach.

Other criteria with which we could make determination of death involved drowning victims who'd been underwater for more than an hour, or pulseless victims who were trapped in a confined space (e.g., a mangled car or a mine shaft) who were unable to be treated by EMS and where extrication time would be greater than fifteen minutes. Patients exhibiting rigor mortis or lividity (when blood settled in the lower portion of the body, causing a purplish discoloration of the skin) were also on the list; we would still need to assess them, though in those cases, it would be to confirm death rather than continue life. "First thing you need to do is make sure the patient has an open airway and assess breathing for thirty seconds to confirm there are no respirations," explained Mrs. Medina. We would also need to confirm there was no cardiac or neurological activity by checking the carotid pulse at the neck and listening for heart sounds for thirty seconds and seeing if the victim's pupils were fixed and dilated when we shined a light in them.

The fact that the L.A. County protocols included a long section on when *not* to treat a patient was a sober reminder of the responsibility of our job. Before she released us for the day, Mrs. Medina said she'd assign our internship spots with a local fire department the following week and that we'd likely start in the field around the middle of June. We all cheered wildly. "You'll also be giving your Grand Rounds presentation next week, so make sure you're ready," she added.

After Mrs. Medina left, we all hung around to discuss our class picture, and once again Lewis championed the idea of taking an "old-school" photo.

"Think of the possibilities," he said excitedly. "We could wear white lab coats and bell-bottoms like that class in 1975."

O'Brien said he wanted to dress up like some students in the August 1976 class picture: "Don a black suit, dangle a cigarette in your hand, and give a suave look that says, 'Paramedic school? . . . Yeah, I did that.'"

"If we imitated the January 1978 class, we could all sport high-waisted pants, plaid shirts, and bushy mustaches," I added.

"Or we could all try to pile into a Volkswagen Bug convertible, like the class from October 1982," Miller suggested.

The options were endless fun. And that didn't even include the 1980s, where we could sport heavy metal hair or the *Miami Vice* look of a V-neck T-shirt and fluorescent blazer.

"I'm in," said Carter.

"Me, too," added Miller.

Other students weren't so sure about the joke. "Is that what we want our legacy to be?" Patel posed.

"True," said O'Brien.

"Aw, come on, guys," said Lewis, "you're only in medic school once in your life."

"Not if you don't pass," said Patel.

A good point.

May

Delivering Babies and
a Do-Not-Resuscitate Order

I spent the remainder of the week immersing myself in the L.A. Country paramedic protocols. I lugged the binder with me everywhere, cracking it open any chance I had—with my morning coffee, on the treadmill at the gym, and even at red lights until the cars behind me honked to hurry up. As I finished reading the last policy, what struck me most was how few words there were on each page. The words were typed in Arial font with a 12-point size.

The rest of the page was—literally—a gray area.

As I closed the protocol book one night, it dawned on me that I'd need to make a big transition from being successful in the classroom to becoming a street-smart paramedic. Who had the secret code to decipher this wide swath of invisible EMS ink? My two paramedic preceptors, whom I'd meet in less than four weeks. I clicked off the light and fell asleep immediately. And then, eight hours later, I helped deliver a baby for the first time.

"You're having another contraction," Julie, an RN at UCLA Medical Center in Santa Monica, told the woman lying in bed 1 of the delivery ward. "Take a deep breath. Hold it in. Round your back and push into your bottom."

The woman in the bed, sweating and pained with contractions, pushed with all her might.

"Great, Edie," coached Julie. "Push! Push! Keep pushing. Almost there . . ."

The labor and delivery ward at the UCLA Medical Center in Santa Monica, known as "the Birthplace," delivered over 1,400 babies a year. For paramedic students who might one day deliver a baby in the field—often in the backseat of a car or at a bus-stop bench, though, not in bright, hotel-like rooms with sofa chair-sleepers—UCLA arranged for each of us to spend a day in an L&D ward, observing the birthing process and practicing hands-on assessment of a newborn.

I'd arrived earlier that morning, at seven, and teamed up with Julie, an Irish gal with fair skin and freckles who balanced the sternness needed during contractions with a sweet bedside manner. "Drop your bag and grab a gown," she'd said to me, "the woman in bed three is about to deliver." That baby had been born covered in meconium—the thick, green stool an infant expels when in distress—so I assisted by using a blue bulb syringe to suction the little girl's mouth and nose, clearing her airway. The second birth was a baby boy born a few weeks premature, who had to be ventilated with a bag-valve mask and rushed to the neonatal intensive care unit (NICU). I helped ventilate him for a few moments in the delivery room and assisted the nurses by pushing the incubator as we hurried to the NICU. Fortunately, both babies—the meconium birth and the preemie—made swift recoveries and the doctors foresaw no long-term complications.

When I returned to the L&D ward, Julie informed me another woman was about to deliver. "Three births in one day," she exclaimed. "You're a white cloud!"

Since she didn't expect any complications, Julie said this birth was all mine. "Right after the doctor catches the baby, she's handing it to you and I want you to perform an assessment and treat anything you find."

As I pulled a yellow gown on over my blue scrubs, Julie reminded me of the importance of drying, warming, and stimulating a newborn. "Keeping them warm is especially important," she said, then she told me a story about some firefighters who once delivered a baby in the field. When the baby arrived, the firefighters discovered their ambulance was out of towels and they had nothing with which to keep the baby warm. "So they took off their shirts to wrap the baby and came into the ER bare-chested in their brush coats," Julie remarked. "Of course, none of us female nurses minded that! And they did a wonderful job."

We hurried to bed 1, where the mom, a thirty-five-year-old woman named Edie, was in the first stage of birth—full dilation. She lay in the bed at a forty-five-degree angle with her lower half covered in sterile blue chux pads.

Julie quickly introduced me. "He's a paramedic with us who'll be assisting today."

Edie smiled. "Nice to meet—" she began, but before she finished, a contraction stole her breath.

"Push-push-push," said the doctor, seated on a little stool at the end of the bed.

The baby was crowning and you could see the tiny head, covered with matted, black hair.

"You're doing great!" said Julie, squeezing Edie's hand.

"Keep pushing," the doctor said, applying gentle counterpressure to the top of the baby's head.

As the contraction ended, Edie rested, collecting her breath. Her husband was evidently stuck in traffic in Culver City on the 405 Freeway. He was desperately trying to arrive in time, but I could tell birth was imminent.

"I think we'll have a baby on our next contraction," the doctor said, looking up at me.

"I'm ready," I replied, crouching slightly like a running back about to receive the handoff.

"I feel another contraction coming on," Edie said, her face wincing in pain.

"Round your back and push into your bottom," encouraged Julie. "Push. Push. Push!"

As Edie pushed, the baby's head appeared, shiny and slick. Then the doctor guided the baby's head down to assist with delivery of the upper shoulder and then back up to help release the lower shoulder. Once the shoulders were free, the rest of the baby followed rapidly.

"We have a boy," the doctor announced with a smile.

"Is he safe?" Edie asked.

"He's beautiful," Julie said. "We're just going to assess him for a moment and then bring him to you."

The doctor suctioned the baby's mouth and nose, cut the cord, and handed him to me. I quickly dried him off, flicked the bottom of his feet, and carried him over to the birthing table with its heat lamp, where Julie waited.

"What next?" she prompted.

"I want to take an Apgar score," I said, continuing to towel him off. "Checking appearance, pulse, grimace, activity, and respirations."

"What do you think his score is?"

The baby's extremities and trunk were pink so I gave him two—the highest score—for appearance. As I listened to his heartbeat, I found it racing like a hummingbird's at 160 beats per minute; and his face wrinkled slightly when I squeezed his toe. "I'll give him twos in pulse and grimace as well," I said.

"How's his activity?" Julie asked. "And respirations?"

The baby's arms and legs weren't limp, but they weren't moving as much as I would've liked, and his respirations seemed a little slow. "For both categories: ones," I remarked. "So his total score is eight out of ten."

When Julie asked how I'd like to fix it, I said I wanted to give the baby oxygen via an infant bag-valve mask.

"I like that you're being proactive," she said, "but try a little more stimulation first."

I flicked the baby's toes once again and squeezed his fingers. "You can be a tad more forceful," Julie said, picking the baby up to flick his feet and rub his back with a towel, "babies are quite resilient."

Julie handed the baby back to me and I imitated her, patting his back, flicking his toes, and rubbing his arms. The baby responded well, moving both arms and legs and emitting his first cry, a beautiful peal of joy.

"I'd rate him a ten now," I said.

"Is he okay?" Edie asked, suddenly worried.

The baby's cry grew stronger. "He wants his mother," Julie said. "So let's swaddle him up and bring him over to her."

I wrapped the baby up in a blanket like a burrito and pulled a blue cap over his head.

As I walked across the room, holding that little life in my hands, I felt the greatest joy and couldn't help but consider that moment as a complement to my experience in the cadaver lab. As paramedics, we'd see dead bodies—stiff and discolored with rigor mortis and lividity—but we would also welcome babies into the world.

And who knew what this little boy's contribution to the world would be, with his happy cry already announcing himself, his arms already reaching into the future?

I would assist with one more delivery that afternoon, a C-section, but presenting Edie with her baby was the highlight of my day. When I arrived at her bedside and handed him to her, you could see all the trials of pregnancy—the morning sickness, weight gain, lower back pain, sleepless nights, and swollen ankles—disappear forever with one glance at her precious new life. Edie was full of excitement, pride, and love for her baby, unable to take her eyes off him.

I finished my third shift at California Hospital that week and was amazed to realize that my time there was already half over. Sometimes it felt like just when I got comfortable with my crew and patient population, I'd be dispatched elsewhere. But maybe that was just life in EMS. And maybe, in the end, comfort is the enemy—because when you're comfortable you may grow complacent, and when you're complacent, you can miss critical signs and symptoms in your patient.

As my clinical shifts progressed, I began to feel as if I'd made strong progress—in taking a quick set of "visual vital signs" when I walked into my patient's room to determine their severity; in methodically checking ABCs and following the flowchart when I assessed a patient; and, as Baxter Larmon had suggested, using all my senses. Could I smell death yet? Initially, I'd assumed Dr. Larmon meant the horrid scent of a decaying body, but now I wondered if he meant something else. Could I catch the scent when death was sitting in the room with a patient—about to strike—and rapidly provide the necessary treatments to reverse it?

I hadn't attempted another intubation. Blame it on my white cloud status—good for my patients, if bad for me gaining experience—but

I was making great strides in other interventions, like injections, 12-lead ECGs, and administering new medications like Lasix (for heart failure) and fentanyl (for pain). On my third shift, Aliyah gave me an impromptu IV clinic. "The bounce, or feel, of a vein is just as important as seeing it," she told me. "If a vein has good bounce, then you know there's a lot of blood moving through." Then she tied an IV tourniquet around my arm and walked me through all the possible IV sites—on top of my hand, on my forearm, in the crux of the elbow, and in the external jugular vein on the side of my neck. "When you need an IV on a critical patient, you go anywhere you can find," she said. "Any port in a storm!" Aliyah also suggested that applying gentle downward pressure on the vein below the injection site with my free hand would help prevent it from rolling and suggested I insert the needle at a shallower angle. "Come in about forty-five degrees, like one of those airplanes landing at LAX," she said. "And once you get a flashback in your catheter, flatten out as you advance and come in for your landing." Thanks to Aliyah's advice, my success rate for IVs improved. I kept track of my IV success like a batting average.

As my clinical shifts sped by, my imminent field internship was increasingly on my mind. I thought of it as my deployment date. To prepare, I chatted with LAFD paramedics anytime they brought a patient in to the ER. When I'd see them wheeling in a patient on their gurney, I'd rush over with the vital sign machine and a kind of barter and trade would take place—I'd get an updated set of vitals and temperature for their patient and they'd give me some insider information on internship.

"Control what you can control," one paramedic said to me. "Have a good attitude. Know your policies. Know your medications. And keep the rig stocked."

"Make decisions and run the call," another advised. "Better to ask for forgiveness than permission."

Another medic told me that if I didn't know something, don't try to make up the answer. "You can't bullshit a fireman," he said. "We know when you're talking out of your ass. So tell them you don't know but that you'll find out." The only advice his partner offered was to raise a hand and extend a forefinger and pinkie, his other fingers forming a muzzle. "Listen like the wolf," he said. "Ears open. Mouth closed."

While a few of my classmates groused during call-ins about their clinical rotations being boring, I enjoyed my time interacting with the patients. There was a body in every bed at California Hospital and a story in every body.

"We all got a beautiful soul, hear what I say!" offered a woman named Jackie who'd come in for elevated blood sugar. "Sometimes it just gets hidden behind the day-to-day."

The main goal in life for another patient, named Willie, who arrived from Skid Row wearing a long black trench coat, was to make everyone smile.

"I'm going to start an IV on you, sir," I said, taking aim.

"Do what you gotta do, brother!" Willie said. Then he hollered to Aliyah as she walked by, "Love the new hairdo, sweetheart!"

Aliyah grinned.

"Aha," Willie shouted triumphantly, "I made you smile!"

It was obvious Willie was a regular at California Hospital—a frequent flyer—but none of the staff seemed to mind.

A moment later, Willie turned to Knox, an ER technician rushing by with the 12-lead ECG machine. "Hey, Knox, how them med school applications coming?"

"I got wait-listed at my top choice and still waiting to hear from the others," Knox replied.

Willie said he was sure it was going to happen for him. "So jes' hang in there, Dr. Knox!"

Knox grinned.

"Aha, I made you smile!"

As I inserted the needle and nailed the IV, Willie's attention was directed back to me. "Nice shot!" he said. "You sure your name ain't Steve Nash?"

Before I could answer—or smile—another patient called me over.

In the next bed, a woman, whose hands shook uncontrollably from acute alcohol withdrawal, said with sad eyes, "Chase your dreams because they won't chase you."

"I was always pursuing property and prestige," another man told me, "but I'd rather be broke and let God provide than be rich and always try to fill that void."

They were the homeless, drug addicts, prostitutes, and ex-convicts of L.A. I wanted to write many off as crazy, but hadn't some of the great prophets preached the same things—love your neighbor, follow your dreams . . . smile? I hadn't expected to find such wisdom and laughter in the ER.

Sadly, this lightness was tempered with tragedy.

On my second shift at California Hospital, two EMTs with a private ambulance wheeled in a seven-month-old baby boy in severe respiratory distress who had a do-not-resuscitate order. The EMTs had been flagged down on the 10 Freeway by the parents who were so desperate for help, they literally tossed the near-dead boy into their arms, so the EMTs raced Code 3 to the nearest hospital, California. When the EMTs called in with a radio report, they were so frantic you could barely hear them above the roar of the sirens—"Seven-month-old . . . Severe shortness of breath and cyanotic . . . DNR."

Mateo and I quickly threw a new set of sheets on a bed in the trauma bay and Aliyah hurried over the crash cart—a locked metal cabinet on wheels that had all the equipment to run a cardiac arrest. Aliyah unlocked the second and fourth drawers—containing pediatric medications, IV solutions, and intubation supplies—and opened the Code Blue log-in binder on top of the cart, readying the sign-in sheet. But I kept wondering why the hell a seven-month-old would have a DNR order. What kind of twisted parents would sign such a form? Just then, the ambulance bay doors opened.

The baby was in his car seat, which the EMTs had smartly seat-belted to the stretcher. The boy wore a small white diaper that clung loosely to his frail body. He was tiny and pale, with a barrel-shaped rib cage and fragile legs that curved toward one another. His eyes had a bluish tint. As he struggled to breathe, his nostrils flared and his arms and legs squirmed.

His parents hurried alongside the gurney. I expected them to be monsters—who signs a DNR on a baby?—but they were a well-dressed, middle-aged couple with red, tear-stained eyes. As they arrived bedside, Aliyah and I moved the baby over and the EMTs again gave a report to the doctor.

"Seven-month-old boy . . . History of brittle bone disease," the EMT said.

As I heard the words "brittle bone disease" suddenly—and tragically—the DNR made sense. The boy had been born with osteogenesis imperfecta, a congenital bone disorder that had no cure. His shortness of breath was likely caused by underdeveloped lungs and the do-not-resuscitate order was in place because chest compressions would shatter the precious boy to pieces. But a DNR kicked in only if the boy stopped breathing, or lost a pulse, and we weren't going to let that happen—not on our watch—so the doctor, Aliyah, Mateo, and I rushed in to take over ventilations, get an IV, and patch him up to the cardiac monitor.

Since I began working as an EMT, people often asked how it felt to watch a patient suffer. It's hard . . . but watching a family grieve is gut-wrenching. As I saw the parents standing bedside that afternoon, watching helplessly as their baby clung to life, my eyes welled with tears and I had to glance away. Our efforts stabilized the boy, but I knew the long-term prognosis wasn't good—most babies born with brittle bone disease don't survive the first year. My shifts in the ER reminded me that life is beautiful, but also brief and very fragile.

I was a little bit of a wreck after leaving the room that day and was on my way to the break room when a voice called out to me.

"Hey, Steve Nash!"

I stopped. "Not now, Willie . . ."

"Are you s-u-u-r-e your name ain't Steve Nash?"

I told him I was certain. "And I'm a Celtics fan."

He extended his hand. "Well, put it here, brother, so am I!"

I couldn't believe this. "You're not a Lakers fan?"

"Hell, nah!" said Willie. "There's no such thing as a Lakers fan; there's just Celtics fans who got lost along the way."

I loved this.

"Aha," he exclaimed, pointing. "I made you smile!"

"Thanks," I said. "I needed that."

I used the baby with the brittle bone disease for my Grand Rounds presentation the following week and asked my classmates all the questions that had initially puzzled me.

"Why would a seven-month-old have a DNR?" I asked.

Naturally, they all thought some form of child abuse—as I had— and when I explained osteogenesis imperfecta, you could hear a pin drop.

"It was a reminder to me that, as paramedics, we never judge a patient or the family until we have all the facts," I said.

Next, I used the case as a jumping-off point to speak about the treatments we might've provided as paramedics and then discussed some of the L.A. County policies regarding DNR orders and dealing with minors.

After everyone presented, Mrs. Medina took the podium. "You guys ready for internship spots?"

Wild applause and cheers filled the room, like Madison Square Garden on NBA draft day. Would the letters above the brim of our form-fitted ball caps read LAFD, LACoFD, Compton, or Long Beach? Few of us had a preference; we were just happy to suit up and play with the pros.

Before she handed out spots, Mrs. Medina reminded us of the field internship schedule—480 to 720 hours under the supervision of two paramedic preceptors who'd had at least two years of field experience themselves. Many of our preceptors would have also attended a one-day UCLA paramedic preceptor course outlining the roles and responsibilities of both preceptor and intern and giving them information on writing evaluations, teaching tactics, scheduling drills, and facilitating hands-on learning. While our preceptors wouldn't receive extra pay for having a "para-puppy" nipping at their heels for twenty to thirty shifts, they would earn some continuing education credits, which helped when they were recertifying their own paramedic license at renewal time. But that was small compensation for the hours preceptors put in, and most simply volunteered to do it because they loved their profession and wanted to help train the next generation of EMS foot soldiers.

Mrs. Medina began by awarding the sponsored students their spots. Naturally, they'd intern with their departments, albeit in different stations. On the surface it seemed like internship would be easier for the sponsored firefighters, but more often than not, the preceptors were harder on their own guys because they had a vested interest in their development.

Next, Mrs. Medina gave spots to the students who'd volunteered with local fire departments and who'd put in special requests. A couple of guys went to Long Beach, Manhattan Beach, or Monrovia, and Carter, along with two other members of the "Compton Clique," would return to "the C-P-T," street slang for Compton, California.

"And for you private students," Mrs. Medina said, "most will intern with L.A. City or L.A. County Fire Department."

O'Brien and I exchanged excited glances across the aisle. Both the Los Angeles Fire Department (also known as the L.A. City Fire Department) and county had large departments with great reputations and over three thousand firefighters and a hundred stations scattered throughout L.A. County. In fact, L.A. County Fire Department had played a large role in putting the paramedic profession on the map: the hit television series from the 1970s, *Emergency!*, had chronicled the adventures of two paramedics from Station 51 of L.A. County Fire Department and had helped introduce the American public to the then-emerging field of paramedicine. As for L.A. City, the department was well-known as one of the best firefighting/EMS agencies in the world, protecting the lives and property of the approximately four million people who lived in America's second largest city.

Despite the similarities, though, the two departments ran medical and trauma calls quite differently. L.A. County responded with a rescue squad—paramedics on a small truck stocked with medical equipment—that met a private ambulance on scene, staffed by two EMTs. If the call was critical, one of the paramedics from the squad would hop onto the private ambulance and treat the patient until they arrived at the hospital. If the patient didn't require any paramedic-level treatments, the paramedics could send them with the private ambulance and wait for another call. L.A. City, on the other hand, operated its own ambulances, staffed by two paramedics who handled the treatment and transport of every patient.

There were pros and cons to each system for a paramedic intern. Interning with L.A. City meant the opportunity to treat and transport all the patients, and a longer continuity of care. However, it also might mean running the basic life support calls for minor complaints and long hours "holding up the wall" at the ER, waiting for a bed for your patient. With L.A. County, you could "ship" patients with mild complaints in a private ambulance, freeing yourself up for more critical calls, but that also meant handing off care to two EMTs you'd never worked with before and a leap of faith that your patient's condition wouldn't deteriorate.

"O'Brien," said Mrs. Medina, scanning the room.

"Here," he said, waving his hand.

"You're going to L.A. City, Station 63 in Venice."

"Yeah, baby!" O'Brien exclaimed.

"It's L.A. City," said Patel. "Watch out!"

"Whatever," O'Brien said coolly. "I'm ready!"

Mrs. Medina returned to her notes. "Miller?"

"Yes, ma'am," he said, nodding.

"You'll be with L.A. County, Station 173 in Inglewood."

"Nice," he said, giving Lewis a high five.

When Mrs. Medina told Patel he'd intern with L.A. City, Station 89 in North Hollywood, Carter noted that he'd better be prepared. "They're hammers at that station!"

Patel said his great cooking skills would help get him through.

And so it went for the next twenty minutes, with Mrs. Medina handing out spots to city and county stations, and the class reacting with a mixture of excitement, expectation, and swagger that, of course, hid our trepidation and uncertainty.

I kept waiting—hoping and praying—for my name to be called, but the day ended abruptly when Mrs. Medina closed her binder and said she was still working on spots for the rest of us. "So just hang in there and I'll let you know next week," she said. "And don't forget about your class picture!"

There were ten of us without internship assignments and, as Mrs. Medina left, we exchanged worried glances. Why us? Had we done something wrong? Were we the runts of the paramedic litter?

Just then, Lewis stood. "As you heard, gentlemen, class pictures next week," he began. "We're definitely going with class A uniforms and suits and ties, but the idea for a throwback old-school picture is still on the table." Lewis promised to e-mail us an update in a few days. "Just to be safe, you might want to think about locating that old mullet wig and fake 'stache."

I knew, however, that whatever photo we did choose—professional or throwback—would have an impressive frame. We had already collected money to have the picture mounted on a stained-wood plaque with a brass plate underneath, bearing everyone's name.

As May ended, I felt our paramedic program rolling like a train toward graduation. But without an internship spot, I felt like I was running alongside the departing train, waiting for the door to open. When I passed her in the hall, Mrs. Medina again assured me she'd have a spot for me next week, but I had a bad feeling in my stomach.

June

In Limbo

"Everyone line up," said Nanci Medina, holding a camera and waving us into place. "Tall people in the back."

June 1, 2011, the thirty-six remaining members of Class 36 stood together on the steps of the Daniel Freeman Hospital for our class pictures, alongside one student from Class 35. He'd had to take a leave of absence from his session due to family issues, so he was joining our class for pictures as well as the clinical and field internship portions of paramedic school.

We'd taken our exam on L.A. County paramedic protocols that morning and I'd scored the third-highest grade in the class. While I was happy to be peaking right before the playoffs, so to speak, I was still worried about not having a spot.

Following our test, Mrs. Medina brought in a surprise guest to lecture us on crime scene investigation. Gil Carrillo was a legendary homicide detective from the Los Angeles County Sheriff's Department who, in 1984 and 1985, had been one of the lead investigators on the infamous "Night Stalker" serial killer case. As paramedics, many of our calls—especially in Los Angeles—would involve crimes such as assault, battery, shootings, and stabbings. Patient care would always be our primary concern, but it was also important to be mindful of the scene and any evidence that might help bring a criminal to justice.

"When you enter a scene, you bring something in with you," Mr. Carrillo said. "And when you leave, you take something out." To assist us with our leave-no-trace ethic, Mr. Carrillo advised us to inform the police if we moved any furniture on scene to, say, clear space for the gurney. If we needed to access the bullet hole in a patient who'd been shot, we should cut around the hole in the clothes and give the cloth to the police for identifying the make and model of the gun. Mr. Carrillo also suggested placing evidence in paper bags instead of plastic, which forms condensation, and not allowing a rape victim to change clothes or shower. "A woman's body *is* the crime scene on a sexual assault," Mr. Carrillo said. "You should try to transport these patients to a hospital that specializes in sexual assault victims and, if possible, have a female partner handle patient care." Before he finished, Mr. Carrillo reminded us of the most important aspect of working in the public service sector, and it wasn't wearing a badge or saying "BSI": "Whether you're a cop or a firefighter, you need a good support system of friends and family and a healthy sense of humor," he said. "Be safe out there, gentlemen, and best of luck."

As Mr. Carrillo finished, Lewis stood. "Give it up for Mr. Gil Carrillo!"

We gave him a rousing standing ovation and Mr. Carrillo was so moved, he called his wife so she could hear and then recorded our cheers to use as his ringtone.

After lunch, we private students changed into our suits and ties, while the sponsored students donned their class A uniforms. Mrs.

Medina snapped a dozen pictures on the steps of the Daniel Freeman Hospital and in front of a large fichus tree on the school grounds that had historically served as a backdrop for many a class picture. Just when Mrs. Medina was about to call it a wrap, Lewis yelled for an outfit change and out came our tie-dyed tank tops, mullet wigs, zoot suits, Elvis shades, white lab coats, and cigarettes.

Initially, I'd been slightly opposed to the idea of an old-school photo, but my clinical shifts—and Mr. Carrillo's lecture that morning—had reminded me that a healthy sense of humor and laughter were as important to an EMS provider as oxygen is to a patient. As paramedics, we would no doubt see gruesome, horrifying scenes and, at times, the darkness of human nature. It was vitally important we not lose sight of the light.

As we reassembled on the steps outside Daniel Freeman Hospital—now with mullets and pompadour wigs blowing in the breeze, Mrs. Medina could hardly contain her laughter long enough to get a good shot.

"On the count of three, say 'BSI'!"

"BSI!" we all hollered with a smile.

"You guys are crazy," she chuckled, snapping pictures.

Following class photos, Mrs. Medina handed out a few more internship spots, but once again, my name wasn't called. As my worries returned—had I done something wrong?— Mrs. Medina again assured me she'd have a spot by the following week. Rather than voice my concerns, I decided to wait another week. I was still in the middle of my clinical rotations, after all, and I had other things to worry about—like finally visualizing the vocal cords and placing an endotracheal tube during my shift in the operating room.

The next day, I was back at UCLA Medical Center in Santa Monica, attempting to intubate a patient.

"Do you see the vocal cords?" asked Dr. Derek Sebold, an anesthesiologist, standing behind me.

"No," I replied, beyond frustrated. I removed my laryngoscope blade, placed an oropharyngeal airway back into the patient's mouth, and asked the nurse on my right to preoxygenate the patient for another attempt.

My day in the operating room hadn't started well. I'd arrived at 6:45 a.m. and checked in with the charge nurse, who immediately pointed to a team of doctors and nurses wheeling a patient in a bed down the hall and said, "They're going to the OR—catch them." I dropped my backpack behind her desk, grabbed my safety glasses and stethoscope, and bounded after them as if trying to hop a boxcar.

"Good morning," I said to the doctor, a man with gray hair, wire-framed glasses, and, it turned out, an English accent. "I'm a paramedic intern. Any chance I can get the tube?"

"I can't see why not," he replied.

In intubation, the Mallampati score is used to predict the difficulty of placing a breathing tube in a patient. The score is based on the height of the mouth and the space between the tongue and the roof of the mouth, along with the amount of open space. A patient who rates as a class 1 or class 2 on the Mallampati score is generally easier to intubate. Patients rated class 3 or 4 are often very difficult.

My first patient that morning was a heavyset man with a thick neck—a Mallampati 4. All I saw when I peered into his mouth was his tongue and the hard palate.

"I can't see the vocal cords," I said to the doctor, handing the laryngoscope blade off to him.

My next patient was, of all things, an opera singer who'd arrived in the OR with explicit instructions for the anesthesiologist not to break his teeth or damage his vocal cords. Maybe not the best candidate for me to learn on (not that I intended to damage anyone's teeth or vocal cords). Plus, the singer was a Mallampati 3. When I looked into his mouth, I spotted the base of the uvula—the dangly flap of tissue in the back of the throat that assists with speech—but the rest of his mouth seemed to be all tongue and teeth. Due to the man's Mallampati score and occupation, I reluctantly handed off the intubation once again. By then, it was late morning and the number of patients going into surgery was fast dwindling. I needed to get at least one intubation, and have the doctors sign my paperwork, or repeat the entire twelve-hour day.

Just then, another patient came rolling down the hall in a hospital bed, pushed by a team of nurses. The doctor leading the procession was an athletic guy in his forties, sporting a high-and-tight military hairdo. I asked if I could try the intubation. "You can't *try*," he replied. "You will *get* the intubation."

I liked Dr. Sebold immediately. He was part of the navy's anesthesiology program, based at the Naval Medical Center in San Diego, and was completing his residency at UCLA Santa Monica. I also favored the intubation prospects of our patient, a lean woman in her late twenties with a long neck who was having knee surgery. As Dr. Sebold sedated her and I placed an OPA in her mouth, I could see she was a class 1 on the Mallampati score. Her uvula and soft palate were entirely visible and I had a lot of room in the oropharynx in which to work. Yet I still couldn't completely visualize her vocal cords on my first intubation attempt, so I removed my blade and told the nurse to continue ventilating her. Dr. Sebold offered me a few helpful hints.

"Everyone has trouble in the beginning," he said. "The key is to change something if you don't get the tube on the first time. If you do the exact same thing over again, you just reinforce your first failure."

As the nurse ventilated the patient, Dr. Sebold discussed my technique. I needed to start by placing my patient's head into the sniffing position to open the airway, which I'd assumed meant a head-tilt, chin-lift maneuver, but Dr. Sebold explained that would actually cut off the airway. "When people sniff, they do this," he said, leaning forward, as if smelling flowers.

"Got it," I said, folding a towel and placing it under the patient's head.

I also needed to insert my laryngoscope blade on the far corner of the mouth instead of at the center. "This prevents the tongue from slipping off to the right," Dr. Sebold explained. "Then you need to lift up on the lower jaw at a forty-five-degree angle, as if you're toasting someone with a glass of champagne."

"I can do that!" I said, with a laugh.

Lastly, he advised me not to lean in so close when I attempted to locate the vocal cords. "Lean back," he said. "When you drive a car, you don't stare at the hood ornament—you look at the road."

"We're at 100 percent O_2," the nurse said. "All ready."

Dr. Sebold glanced over at me. "Ready for another attempt?"

"Let's do it," I said, turning to the nurse. "Stop bagging, please, and remove the OPA."

On this attempt, I allowed myself a solid five seconds to sweep the tongue out of the way. Along with correct head positioning, I decided a good tongue sweep would set me up for success. Next I inserted my laryngoscope on the far right corner of the cheek, caught the tongue in the curve of my blade, and gently displaced it to the far left of the mouth, being mindful not to break any teeth. Once the tongue was clear, I inserted my blade into the vallecula (a depression behind the root of the tongue that traps saliva) and lifted up. As I did, I saw the epiglottis, the flap of elastic cartilage that prevents food and water from entering the trachea.

"Good! Now lift a little higher," Dr. Sebold coached, "and tell me what you see."

"Vocal cords!" I exclaimed joyfully.

They were shiny with saliva and lined the trachea like a white picture frame. I glanced up at the nurse. "ET tube, please."

The nurse handed me the tube and I quickly inserted it. As the tiny balloon cuff at the end of the tube passed between the vocal cords, I quickly removed my laryngoscope blade, used a syringe to inflate the distal cuff, and instructed the nurse to connect the bag-valve mask to the tube and deliver a breath.

"No sounds over the stomach," I announced, listening with my stethoscope.

The nurse delivered two more breaths.

"And I've got clear bilateral breath sounds and good chest rise," I said.

"Now what?" asked Dr. Sebold.

I told him we would secure the tube in the mouth with a plastic "tube tamer" and further confirm placement by monitoring the patient's carbon dioxide levels with an end-tidal CO_2 detector.

"What levels are we looking for?"

"Between 35 and 45mmHg," I said.

"What if the number's below 35?"

"We'd slow our ventilatory rate because the patient needs more carbon dioxide."

"And if the number's above 45mmHg?"

"We speed up."

Dr. Sebold shook my hand. "Congratulations on your first intubation!"

"Thanks!" I replied excitedly. Successfully intubating my first live patient felt like making the game-winning shot at the buzzer.

I shadowed Dr. Sebold for the remainder of that afternoon, successfully intubating two more patients, a Mallampati class 2 and class 3. I was thrilled but, as I emerged into the bright sunshine of Sixteenth Street in Santa Monica, I wondered how intubation would go in the field setting—when my patients hadn't been fasting for twelve hours before the procedure; hadn't had a chest X-ray to confirm that their lungs were clear; and weren't served up on a table under the bright lights of the operating room. How would it be to perform an intubation on a middle-aged man lying pulseless on his living room floor as his children looked on?

I had to be ready.

As June arrived, I finished at California Hospital and worked my first three shifts at St. Joseph's in Burbank. There, I bandaged a man with a deep puncture wound on his forearm from a pit bull; irrigated the eye of an eight-year-old girl who'd been burned with a marshmallow at a bonfire; and applied oxygen to a four-year-old boy who'd accidentally eaten his mother's pot brownies. Another man had been wheeled into the ER with a Viagra-induced persistent erection.

"How do you treat that?" I asked Kelly, a blond nurse who loved country music and described herself as "a California gal with a Southern heart."

"Viagra is a nitrate, so it dilates vessels," she replied, quizzing me, "so what could we give?"

"We need vasoconstriction," I said. "I'd say epinephrine, but that's contraindicated because it could shut off all blood supply and perfusion in the area."

"Pseudoephedrine," said Kelly, holding up a syringe. "Want to work on your injection skills?"

"Thanks, but that medication is out of my scope of practice," I said.

Kelly laughed. "Okay, then go start an IV for me on bed six."

"With pleasure," I said, grabbing an IV start kit.

I wasn't sure if it was hospital policy or simply doctors unwilling to cede procedures to paramedic interns, but either way, I wasn't allowed to intubate patients at St. Joe's. And since St. Joe's didn't have the busy pulse of California Hospital—where assault, stabbing, and "GSW" (gunshot wound) victims arrived almost daily—

I focused instead on my patient assessment and IV skills. I'd enter a room, imagining I was a paramedic arriving on scene, and perform a quick assessment to decide if a patient was a "load and go" or a "stay and play." Next, I'd decide which hospital I'd transport the person to and what treatments I could provide under the prior-to-base-contact protocols outlined in Policy 806.

"Good afternoon, sir," I said to one sixty-five-year-old man who'd arrived at St. Joe's because he'd had a seizure.

"Go to hell," he said, his face turning red.

His wife, a polite, soft-spoken woman, told me he had a history of dementia, ever since he'd gotten a traumatic brain injury in a fall a few years before. I'd heard that patients with dementia often presented in one of two ways—the friendly dementia and the other kind.

I asked the man what had brought him into the ER today.

"I said go to hell, you motherfucker!"

"Simon! Be nice to this young man," his wife said, likely wondering where the man she'd married had disappeared to.

I tried to continue. "Do you have any pain, sir?"

"Listen, if you don't get the hell out of here right now . . ." Simon was growing more agitated, so, following the maxim of "Do no harm," I thanked his wife for their time and moved on. Paramedics often dealt with altered, agitated patients, and had I encountered this couple in the field, I knew that even if Simon wouldn't talk to me, I could've obtained a patient history from his wife to determine if his agitation was a new development. Had there been any recent trauma? If I was on the ambulance, I'd do a full workup on him—vitals, ECG, blood sugar—and perhaps consider a sedative such as midazolam (Versed) or Ativan to calm him.

The patient in the next room was a forty-three-year-old male who said he'd had an allergic reaction to eating a steak sandwich. Hives dotted his back with red spots. I quickly checked his ABCs to rule out anaphylactic shock—ensuring that his throat wasn't swelling, he wasn't short of breath, and his blood pressure was stable.

"What would you do for him?" inquired Kelly.

"Benadryl. Slow IV push," I said.

"No epinephrine?"

I told her the patient was denying any shortness of breath and his blood pressure, at 140/88, was within normal limits. "But if his symptoms worsened I'd consider epinephrine via an IM injection to his deltoid."

"Strong work!" she congratulated me.

The next patient, a ninety-year-old man who'd arrived from a convalescent home, had all the symptoms of septic shock—a recent infection, systolic blood pressure below 100, a temperature and pulse above 100, along with rapid shallow breathing. The cause of his infection was likely the stage 4 pressure ulcer on his hip that was dripping a yellowish ooze. I decided that, in the field, I'd put him on high-flow oxygen, lay him flat—to help with blood pressure—start an IV, and give him normal saline, assessing his lungs often so as not to overload him on fluid; and I'd transport him rapidly to the hospital, where he'd likely have his bloodwork done, receive additional fluid and antibiotics via a central IV line, and perhaps be intubated.

My shifts at St. Joe's were enjoyable. Though I felt stuck in limbo, still waiting to be assigned a field internship spot, I improved my IV skills and patient rapport. But the relatively quiet pace of St. Joe's changed on the evening of my fourth shift, when LAFD paramedics radioed in to say they were transporting a fifty-eight-year-old woman in severe distress. I couldn't hear additional details above the roar of sirens but I did catch the words "vomiting" and "blood."

"What do you think it could be?" Kelly asked as we readied a bed in the trauma bay.

"GI bleed, stomach ulcer, cancer," I said, "or a tear in the esophagus, trauma . . ."

Kelly said she knew the medics well. "They're at the top of the game. If they're worried, it's serious." She added that she thought the patient might be suffering from esophageal varices, a life-threatening condition that occurs when blood flow to the liver becomes obstructed by scar tissue or a clot. Seeking a way around the blockage, blood seeps into smaller vessels, where it collects, building like a water balloon until one day it pops.

Lucy, another nurse, peeked her head in. "They're here."

Kelly and I hurried into the hallway to find the paramedics wheeling the woman in. She was ghost-pale and projectile vomiting bright red blood with every breath, and she wore a look of impending doom on her face. A firefighter off the engine hurried alongside the gurney, catching the vomit in an emesis bag about to overflow.

"Where to?" asked the lead paramedic.

"Bed two," Kelly replied, pointing.

"What's her medical history?" the ER doctor asked, falling in line with us.

"Liver cirrhosis. Recovering alcoholic," the medic said.

Just then, the woman's eyes rolled into the back of her head and her body slumped.

"She's crashing," yelled Kelly.

When we arrived in the trauma bay, we transferred her into a bed. Lucy rushed in to suction the woman's mouth with a rigid-tip suction catheter, and Kelly and another nurse were at each arm, attempting to start an IV. As hospital personnel rushed in, the room quickly became cramped with nurses, doctors, and respiratory therapists.

"She needs to be intubated now! Get a transfusion of packed red blood cells started and we need to plug the esophagus and stop the bleeding with a Blakemore tube until we can get her into surgery," the doctor called out. "And I need everyone who's not directly involved in patient care out of the room right now!"

I was pushed out into the hallway and a nurse closed the curtain in the trauma bay, blocking my view. "You will learn to smell death," Dr. Larmon had said—and there it was, in the clotted blood pouring out of that woman's mouth; in the wide, terrified look in her eyes and her fading breath. I hated the scent and decided, as a paramedic, I'd always do everything in my power to prevent it.

Mrs. Medina's "Intro to Field" lecture later that week marked a critical point in the paramedic program—our last scheduled session at school. Class 36 wouldn't assemble again as a group until graduation day . . . assuming we made it that far.

Mrs. Medina started by explaining the format of internship. "You'll complete at least twenty shifts but it's common for that to be extended to twenty-five or thirty shifts if there are problem areas or if interns haven't gotten the critical calls they need to sign off on certain skills." Over the course of internship, we'd need at least forty advanced life support "contacts," meaning we performed an intervention above the EMT level, such as pushing a medication, starting an IV, or intubating a patient. We would record each patient's age, sex, and chief complaint on a daily evaluation form, along with the treatments we provided, and our preceptors would grade us and add comments. The calls would be graded with a 1, 2, or 3. A "1" meant we had "failed to perform." Borderline, inconsistent calls were awarded a "2," and "3" meant we were competent.

In addition to daily forms, our preceptors would give us major evaluations on our seventh, fourteenth, and twentieth shifts. Along with running calls, we would also be required to present a proficiency drill every shift to the crew. The topics of proficiency drills could include protocols, ambulance inventory, medications, or how to perform a specific treatment like a needle decompression.

"But your main job is to run calls," Mrs. Medina said, "keep the ambulance stocked, and study."

To pass our internship, we'd have to receive "3s" in every category on our daily evaluations—scene management, patient assessment, communication, leadership, and treatment skills. If 90 percent of success in life is about showing up, during field internship that meant showing up early. "If you're early, you're on time," Mrs. Medina told us. "If you're on time, you're late. And if you're late, don't even bother showing up."

Mrs. Medina told us a story about an intern who'd arrived late for his very first shift, only to see the ambulance and engine taking off to a call without him. "He hadn't even run a call yet and already he had to dig himself out of a very deep hole."

Mrs. Medina said one key to success in the field was putting the firefighters on the engine to work by delegating tasks to them such as checking vital signs and blood sugar, hooking up oxygen, and patching a patient up to the heart monitor. "It's up to you: Do you want more hands on deck? Or more eyes standing around watching you?"

O'Brien leaned over and said he wasn't so sure about delegating tasks when it came to the LAFD. "My friend asked one of the firefighters on the engine to get him a blood pressure during his internship," he whispered, "the guy just looked at him and laughed."

Mrs. Medina concluded her lecture by reminding us that we were guests in the firehouse and we should be respectful at all times—and that it was also a tradition to cook a good dinner for your crew on your last shift as a way of saying thank you. "Internship is going to be hard and your preceptors are going to nitpick the hell out of you," she warned, "but if you get through this, you deserve to be paramedics. Good luck, and be safe out there."

After Mrs. Medina left, we gathered around Lewis and Carter. As a firefighter with Santa Monica and a volunteer with Compton Fire Department, they'd witnessed a bunch of guys go through internship before and seemed to have valuable insider information about this unique paramedic rite of passage.

The general consensus of our class was that we'd be like "boots," slang for the lowest-ranking, most probationary firefighter with LAFD. But Carter and Lewis immediately squashed that idea.

"A boot?" said Carter. "You'll be like a used tennis shoe."

"Not even that," added Lewis. "A broken flip-flop!"

For the next five minutes, they schooled us on internship, with Carter providing the commentary and Lewis the color.

Carter: "Never put your hands in your pockets."

Lewis: "Just sew 'em shut!"

Carter: "Keep your hair short."

Lewis: "Shave it off right now!"

Carter: "Never sit down."

Lewis: "Unless you're in the bathroom or at dinner."

Carter: "Eat your meals fast."

Lewis: "Shovel that shit down."

Carter: "Always be the last one up to bed every night."

Lewis: "And first up in the morning."

Carter: "Bring ice cream on your orientation shift."

Lewis: "Dreyer's—not Breyers—gentlemen!"

Carter: "Don't speak unless spoken to."

Lewis: "Be seen, but not heard."

Carter: "Never miss a call."

Lewis: "Sleep on the bottom step of the staircase, or in the ambulance if necessary."

Carter: "No texting on duty."

Lewis: "Just smash your cell phone right now."

Carter: "Don't miss a shift."

Lewis: "Shows 'em you're not committed."

Carter: "If they ask if you want to work for their department, say no—even if it's your dream job."

"Why?" I interrupted.

"Because then they'll be extra tough on you!" Carter explained. "Why make a hard thing harder?"

"Tell them you want to be a flight medic or something," added Lewis.

We all nodded, taking mental notes.

"And the last thing," Carter said. "If they give you advice, don't ever say, 'Well, in paramedic school, they taught us to . . .'"

"Oh, hell no!" howled Lewis.

I realized Lewis and Carter had neglected to mention one very important thing. "What about saying 'BSI' and 'scene safe'?" I asked.

Lewis burst out laughing and Carter looked at me like I was crazy. "If you say 'BSI' on scene with LAFD they are going to call in a helicopter and fly your ass back to Daniel Freeman!"

So there it was. But without an internship, I was still unable to put any of these concepts to use.

I stopped in Mrs. Medina's office on my way out to find out what the latest was on my internship spot. Almost all of my classmates had their assignments already, and most were starting in the field the following week, so I was hopeful that there might be some good news for me.

There wasn't.

"We're still trying," she said. "I'm waiting to hear back from a couple of captains, so just hold tight."

My heart sank. With no more classroom meetings and just one ER shift remaining, I felt all the momentum of the last six months screech to a halt. Would I finish internship to graduate on time? Was I still a member of Class 36?

When two more weeks passed and I still didn't have a spot, I sent an e-mail to Heather Davis, the program director, and Mrs. Medina, hoping for an answer.

By then, I'd finished my ER rotations and had also spent a day in the pediatric intensive care unit (PICU) at Long Beach Memorial. There, I'd suctioned the endotracheal tube of a fourteen-year-old boy who'd been critically injured in a car crash; checked vital signs on a three-month-old baby girl who'd suffered cardiac arrest and had miraculously been revived; and listened to a grieving family say their last words to their fifteen-year-old son who was brain-dead after being hit on his bike by a drunk driver. The PICU was in some ways the saddest place on earth, and I walked out into the bright sunshine that afternoon with a heavy heart. But it was also the most spirited place, and I couldn't help but feel forever inspired by those kids. They were all critical, and yet not one of them focused on their injury or illness. Instead, they chose to focus on the Get Well cards their class-mates had sent; the ice cream and Nintendo games the nurses brought; the cartoons they could watch on endless repeat; the friends and family who visited; and all the dreams—*I want to be a teacher! A professional baseball player! An astronaut!*—they had for when they felt better. Rather than lament being saddled with urinary tubes, endotracheal tubes, or oxygen masks, they chose to focus on all the beauty and possibility still left in the world—they chose joy.

As my clinical shifts ended, I tried to stay productive by returning to school to practice scenarios with another student who was also waiting for a spot. But we breezed through all the mock emergencies with ease. Classroom scenarios had little left to teach us and we craved the concrete knowledge that only comes from running calls on the street.

I was worried about losing momentum; about the possibility of not being finished with internship by my scheduled graduation date; and about UCLA's use of merit in assigning stations, and what it meant that fellow students with lower GPAs had received field assignments ahead of me. After sending my e-mail to Ms. Davis and Mrs. Medina, I received replies from both immediately that helped set my mind at ease. Ms. Davis explained the situation in more detail: budget cuts to LACoFD and LAFD had created gaps in EMS personnel and assignments. Many of the smaller departments, having faced similar problems, now had paramedic assessment fire engines—instead of ambulances—which had no extra seats for an intern. Class 36 also had a high number of private students, and since two other paramedic programs in L.A. were also sending students into field internship at the same time, those students were snagging some of the spots usually reserved for UCLA students.

Ms. Davis echoed Mrs. Medina, and explained that the school had never lacked internship spots before, so they'd never needed a system for awarding spots. In the past, they'd simply matched the department requirements, as well as preceptor and student personalities, in assigning a spot. Ms. Davis promised UCLA had "all hands on deck," trying to rectify the shortage of internship assignments, and added that the school had just gotten commitments for four spots with departments in L.A. County. Ms. Davis said she expected Mrs. Medina might contact me with an internship assignment as early as the following day.

To my great relief, she did.

The next afternoon, I was studying L.A. County policies at a

Starbucks in El Segundo when my cell phone lit up with Mrs. Medina's number.

"Hello?" I said excitedly, hurrying outside.

Mrs. Medina said she'd found me a spot. "You'll be with the Los Angeles Fire Department, Station 38 in the neighborhood of Wilmington."

I was thrilled. "Thank you so much!"

I had no idea where Wilmington was, but Mrs. Medina explained that it was located in the Harbor area of L.A., framed by Long Beach, San Pedro, Harbor City, and Carson. "LAFD staffs three rotating platoons," she explained, "so you'll work twenty-four hours on, twenty-four hours off. Twenty-four on, twenty-four off. Twenty-four on, and then four days off."

"Got it," I said, scribbling notes.

Mrs. Medina said I'd start in two weeks. "July tenth is your orientation shift and you'll begin in the field on the fifteenth."

I was so excited, I almost hung up before asking about my preceptors.

Mrs. Medina told me I'd be with Tim Hill and Eddie Higgins. Tim had graduated from Daniel Freeman in 1996 and had worked at Station 9 in downtown L.A. for a number of years before transferring to Station 38. Eddie had worked as a paramedic in San Bernardino County before getting hired by LAFD and had won a number of performance excellence awards. "Both are great paramedics," Mrs. Medina said. "You'll learn a lot from those guys."

The minute Mrs. Medina assigned me a spot, I felt my momentum return . . . in high gear. I went from having a few weeks of no demands on my time to having a thousand things to do—learn everything possible about the Los Angeles Fire Department, the Wilmington neighborhood, the Lifepak 15 cardiac monitor and the Ferno heavy-lift gurney LAFD used in their ambulances, and all the hospitals in their area. I also had to get sized and fitted for a station uniform, study up on protocols, plan my proficiency drills, and put a new coat of black polish on my boots.

To brush up on medication administration and my IV skills, I scheduled an extra shift at California Hospital that Saturday night. As always, the hospital was busy, and that night the ER resembled a Halloween party even more than usual. With California Hospital's close proximity to the Staples Center and convention center, the clientele changed with the event—Lakers games, country music concerts, marijuana and porn expos. That evening, an anime convention had set up shop at the convention center to celebrate the popular Japanese animation style. Thus, I was starting IVs on patients wearing purple kimonos, ninja shoe covers, black fishnet stockings, white formal dresses, long cloaks, and knee-high socks.

But whenever LAFD brought someone in, I'd take a few moments to pump the paramedics for information about my new station and preceptors.

"Wilmington is the hood of the South Bay," one medic told me. "It's the only place in America where some of the projects have an ocean view."

Another firefighter highlighted all the target hazards in the area: "You've got highways, the harbor, oil refineries, junkyards, and, of course, all the gangbangers."

When I asked about Tim and Eddie, I got the sense both men were held in very high regard within the department.

"Tim is a great medic," a firefighter said. "And a pretty laid-back guy. Likes to fish and surf."

"Eddie's great, too," his partner added, "but he can be high-strung and harsh. Listen to what he says—not how he says it."

In between IVs and soliciting info, I also spent some time in the radio booth with Mateo, one of the head nurses, listening to paramedics call in with their radio reports. Calls arrived for assaults, overdoses, seizures, and stabbings. Sitting there listening, you'd swear the Battle for L.A. was raging right outside the ER doors.

And maybe it was.

By eleven p.m., I was exhausted and my head throbbed painfully. Mateo ordered me to go home and get some sleep. "You've got internship to prepare for!"

I thanked him. Grabbed my backpack and said good-bye to Aliyah and the rest of the nursing team and then hopped in my car, heading south on the 110 Freeway. The freeway was dark and strangely empty and you could hear the roar of your tires in the concrete grooves. From downtown, the 110 Freeway travels nineteen miles south before ending abruptly near a neighborhood of industrial junkyards, trucking firms, oil refineries, and weekly motels, a forsaken place called Wilmington. *The best way out is through.* I'd been saying it for months, and now I was about to live it.

Gulp.

Three | *Field Internship*

A man cannot have better fortune than to be able, nor a better temper than be willing, to save many.

—*Cicero*

Looking back now on the days I spent riding ambulances full time, I realize they were the best days I have known in medicine. They were days of adventure and challenge and the shared pride in having done a tough job well.

—*Dr. Nancy Caroline*

July

Field Internship Begins

Fire Station 38, which serves the 9.1 square miles of Wilmington, wasn't LAFD's busiest station, but it wasn't exactly a sleepy hollow, either. With sixteen murders in 2011—an average of one per 1.7 square miles—and dozens of other assault and gunshot wound victims, Wilmington would finish the year ranked as the twenty-fifth deadliest area (out of L.A. County's 272 neighborhoods) by the *L.A. Times* Homicide Report.

"You're going to Belligerent City," Rod Hillerts, a retired LAFD firefighter, told me. "You'll see it all there—druggies, gangbangers, drunks."

Rod had worked for LAFD for twenty years, a few months of which he'd spent at Station 38 in Wilmington. He said "38s" was a good station that a lot of firefighters wanted to work in. "The firefighters tend to be older and there aren't a lot of hotheads there."

Prior to my orientation shift, I'd arranged to have dinner with Rod and Anna Nilssen, herself a retired firefighter/paramedic with Orange County Fire Authority, to pick their brains about internship.

Rod and Anna were a couple who lived a few houses down from my parents in San Clemente, California, and they had generously agreed to give me their time to help me prepare.

"What battalion is Station 38 in?" Rod quizzed me.

"Six," I replied confidently. I'd spent the last few days studying everything I could find about the department, neighborhood, and local hospitals.

"How many fire stations are in Battalion 6?"

"Ten."

When Anna asked me what hospitals were near Wilmington, I was able to name Kaiser Medical Center in Harbor City, Harbor-UCLA in Torrance, and Torrance Memorial, along with St. Mary and Little Company of Mary and Long Beach Memorial.

Rod smiled, taking a swill of his margarita. "You've done your homework. That's good."

Anna told me to never lose sight of my drug box. "People will steal it right out from under you. They want the narcotics," she explained. "I used to sit on mine on scene."

When I asked Rod and Anna about the craziest calls they'd seen, Anna told me about a mother who'd dressed her two daughters up in their Sunday best, then shot them both in the head. "I'll never forget the father's guttural scream when he found out his daughters were gone," she replied sadly. Rod didn't tell me a specific story; he just grew silent, dropped his eyes, and shook his margarita glass slightly to shift the ice. "After a career in the fire service, the thing that amazes me most is the cruelty one human being can inflict on another."

The sun had set by then and the palm trees threw starfish-shadows on the concrete.

"Any last words of wisdom before I start?" I asked.

"Do your best, and don't be cocky," Anna replied.

Rod told me to really show the guys at the station that I wanted to learn. "And be worried if they *don't* make fun of you!"

Fire Station 38 occupied a large, square, two-story building on I Street, across from a historic hotel called the Don (now senior apartments) and next to a small park where, on hot afternoons, local guys gathered to sip beer out of brown paper bags and sleep in the shade. Wilmington Jewelry & Loan—billed as "one of the world's largest pawn shops"—sat just a stone's throw away on Avalon Boulevard, the north–south boulevard that divides Wilmington in more ways than one. The Eastside Wilmas street gang claimed the neighborhood east of Avalon, and the Westside Wilmas claimed, you guessed it, the west. Both street gangs sported shaved heads, tattoos, and sagging pants; they all prayed to the same God, listened to the same music, rooted for the Dodgers and Lakers, celebrated the same holidays, and spoke the same native language. They were all young Hispanics struggling to carve out an existence for themselves and their families in arguably America's roughest city. But just because they lived on separate sides of the street, they also sprayed bullets at one another.

Historically, Fire Station 38 was staffed by twelve firefighters who responded to incidents on a ladder truck, fire engine, and rescue ambulance. However, a few months prior to my arrival, the station had lost its ladder truck due to budget cuts. Now only six firefighters staffed Station 38, four on the engine and two paramedics on the ambulance.

Standing at the station door with a gallon of Cookies 'N Cream ice cream under my arm—Dreyer's, not Breyers—I rang the doorbell at 9:15 a.m. on July 10.

A moment later, the door opened and a firefighter greeted me. He was a man in his fifties with sandy blond hair and blue eyes. He wore his station uniform and appeared freshly showered.

"Tim Hill," he said, extending a hand. "Your preceptor."

I quickly introduced myself. Thanked him for precepting me and handed him the ice cream.

"Thanks," he replied. "Let's introduce you to the rest of the crew."

I followed Tim into the kitchen, where the guys on the engine sat at a long table, chomping on breakfast burritos. They all wore navy blue station uniforms and leapt to their feet the moment they saw me.

"Welcome," said Captain Turner. "Great to have you here and we look forward to working with you."

Captain Turner had worked for LAFD as a firefighter and paramedic for over twenty years and also taught at the drill tower where they trained new firefighter recruits.

The rest of the crew was equally accomplished. Bryan had played professional baseball prior to joining LAFD. Nick, the engineer, had worked for years as a firefighter and paramedic before being promoted, and Carlos had been with the department longer than Captain Turner. They were all warm and welcoming, but I wondered: where was Eddie?

Captain Turner invited me to sit. "Tell us a little bit about yourself."

I spoke briefly about growing up in New Hampshire, attending college in Seattle, my prior work experience, and my journey into EMS.

"Why do you want to be a paramedic?" Nick asked, placing a cup of coffee in my hand.

All the firefighters were seated around the table now—an early morning interview panel of five.

"I think helping people is one of the things that makes me happiest," I began, my feet tapping under the table with a nervous energy. "As paramedics, I think we have the opportunity to really change the outcome of an emergency and make a difference. I think working is—"

Just then, a voice called out from the back of the room. "Anytime he starts a sentence with 'I think,' don't believe him . . ."

I turned to see a tall and wiry guy with a wad of tobacco in his lower lip and both thumbs tucked into his belt. The way he leaned against the double doors leading to the apparatus floor reminded me of Paul Newman in the classic western *Hud*.

"That's Eddie," Bryan replied.

I immediately stood and shook his hand.

"Come on," Eddie said. "Let's show you the ambulance."

Rescue Ambulance 38 (RA 38) was a Type I ambulance with a Braun Northwest North Star module mounted onto a Dodge Ram light truck chassis. The rig had arrived only a few weeks ahead of me and, with its bright red paint, diamond plate aluminum running boards, LED intersection lights, and speakers in the grille, looked like the paramedic equivalent of something on MTV's show *Pimp My Ride*.

Eddie threw open the back doors, revealing the patient compartment. It had the sterile, gray, bright feel of an ER. Recessed lights on the ceiling illuminated a red Ferno gurney, situated on the left side of the patient compartment. A captain's chair sat at the head of the gurney in the back of the ambulance, next to a small console with a computer screen displaying dispatch information. To the right, a long gray bench seat (filled with cardboard arm and leg splints, as well as a traction splint used for midshaft femur fractures) ran parallel to the gurney. The rest of the patient compartment was filled with medical equipment of every size and shape—oxygen, masks, needles, angiocatheters, bags of IV fluid, medications, trauma dressings, and soft restraints. It wasn't so much an ambulance as an emergency room that had been shrink-wrapped to fit on four tires. Eddie climbed in, snagging the captain's chair. Tim grabbed the bench seat, and I slid in next to him.

"First thing to do when you come in in the morning is put your safety equipment on the rig and get a report from the off-duty crew," Eddie explained.

"Find out if we're down any backboards, narcotics, or oxygen bottles, and what the fuel status is," added Tim.

"Yeah, 'cause if we need something on a run and it's not there, guess who we're coming after?" warned Eddie.

"Yes, sir," I replied.

After my morning report, I'd take inventory of all the equipment on the ambulance, checking every last detail, right down to the expiration dates on all the medications and number of electrodes in the back pocket of the cardiac monitor. "That'll take a few hours if it's done right," said Tim. "And then you're welcome to help out with station duties or put on a proficiency drill." The drills were suggested to run up to thirty minutes in length and could include props, drawings, or diagrams.

Eddie pulled out a copy of the Field Internship Daily Performance Record. I'd record all the calls and treatments each day and Eddie and Tim would grade my performance and write comments. Specifically, they would assess my scene management, treatment decisions, communication, leadership, and practical skills and, as Mrs. Medina had mentioned, would give me major evaluations on my seventh, fourteenth, and twentieth shifts.

"If he lasts that long," said Eddie with a smirk.

I was to wear my station uniform at all times during the day. At night, however, I could wear my blue UCLA Paramedic Education Program T-shirt, along with yellow turnouts, boots, and a brush coat.

"What would you say is your biggest weakness?" Eddie asked.

Since my previous EMT experience had been largely in controlled environments, like a ski resort and the clinical setting, I told them that I wanted to improve my scene management, particularly in the context of running calls with the fire department. "I'm excited to learn from you both," I said, "and I'm willing to do whatever it takes to grow in this area."

Eddie nodded, spitting tobacco juice into his receptacle of choice—a disposable EMS exam glove.

When Tim asked what my greatest strength as an EMT was, I told him I felt very confident in patient assessment. "I've worked hundreds of hours with patients, both in the clinical setting and the field, so I feel very confident there."

"We'll see about that," Tim said with a tone of voice that told me I had no idea what the hell was in store for me.

Eddie agreed. "The field is totally different from the clinical setting," he said. "Doctors and nurses in the ER have it easy because the chief complaint and initial treatments have been served up by the paramedics."

Before they let me go, Eddie had one last question: "Do you want to work for LAFD one day?"

I recalled the advice from Carter and Lewis to keep my mouth shut. "Why make a hard thing harder?" Lewis had said, knowing it would make our preceptors harder on us. But not being honest didn't feel right.

"Yes, sir," I said, looking at both Tim and Eddie. "I'd be honored to work for LAFD."

Eddie chuckled, as if I'd just scattered the last shovelful of dirt atop my grave. "You shouldn't have said that," he said, confirming what my classmates had warned. He spit again into the glove. "Now we're going to be extra hard on you!"

Maybe so, but I wasn't looking for anyone to take it easy on me, either. I glanced over at Eddie, hunched forward in the captain's chair, tapping his foot nervously, his elbows on his knees. And then at Tim, leaning back causally on the bench seat with his legs extended onto the gurney. Where Eddie was full of coiled energy and poised to strike, Tim was laid-back and calm. They were like red and black jumper cables—Eddie supplied the spark and Tim the grounding—to kick-start my medic motor.

Tim shook my hand. "See you July fifteen at zero six hundred."

I left Fire Station 38 that afternoon and spent the next five days prepping for my first shift. I picked up my station uniform at Galls public safety and apparel store in Westchester and checked the UCLA paramedic patch on the left arm and spelling on my nameplate. I reviewed Policy 506, about which patients required immediate transport to a trauma center—*patients with penetrating injuries to the head, neck, or torso; amputations proximal to the wrist or ankle; falls from heights greater than 15 feet . . .*

I recited medications in my mind: *Morphine. For moderate to severe pain. Slow IV push. Titrate to pain relief; may repeat one time. Contraindications include systolic blood pressure less than 100; allergy, head injury, altered patients, low respiratory rate . . .*

I got a haircut, and as the barber tucked a white towel into my shirt collar, he asked, "How would you like your hair today?"

"Number two clippers on the sides and back and a half inch off the top, please," I replied.

He asked if I was going to a wedding.

"Paramedic internship."

"I'm sorry," he replied, clicking on the razor.

I spread out all my equipment on my bed and took inventory one last time. Stethoscope. *Check.* Penlight. *Check.* Blood pressure cuff. *Check.* Safety glasses. *Check.* Clipboard. *Check.* Daily evaluation forms. *Check.* Sleeping bag. *Check.* Station uniform. *Check.* UCLA T-shirt and ball cap. *Check.* Toiletries. *Check.*

The morning of my first day, I awoke at four thirty. Showered. Shaved. Got dressed. Had breakfast. And then found myself driving south on the 110 Freeway in the predawn darkness, en route to Wilmington, wondering just what the city would serve up for me on my first day.

I arrived to find Station 38 sealed up like a fortress. All the lights were off and the doors locked. I parked on the street and pondered my options: Did I ring the doorbell and risk waking up (and maybe pissing off) the firefighters? Or did I wait, and risk being deemed late? Why hadn't Mrs. Medina covered this? *Oh well*, I thought, readying my hand to push the doorbell. *The best way out is through*.

Just then, I heard a truck turn down I Street. It was Tim, driving a Jeep with surf racks. The top was down and it rode on big, Baja-ready tires with a license plate frame that said, "Respect the Beach."

Of course.

"You can pull your car into the fenced-in lot next to the station," he said, rolling up.

"I'm fine on the street," I replied, not wanting to overstep my bounds.

"Come on," he said, a little annoyed. "It's Wilmington."

Despite his laid-back attitude and our shared affinity for riding waves, Tim made it immediately clear there wasn't going to be any buddy-buddy surfer shit between us—at least not until internship was over. "Get a report from the off-going crew and get started on inventory," he said, handing me a yellow brush coat, a blue fire helmet—designating me a single-function paramedic intern—and a bulletproof vest.

LAFD began requiring personnel to wear bulletproof vests on gunshot wound and assault calls after Scott Miller, an apparatus operator with LAFD, got shot in the cheek while en route to a call during the Rodney King riots of 1992. The bullet traveled down Miller's neck before lodging itself in his windpipe. Thanks to the fast actions of his crew—who stopped the bleeding and diverted the truck to Cedars-Sinai Medical Center—and the strength of

Miller's strong spirit and supportive family, he survived the injury and later worked in the Fire Prevention Bureau, serving the San Fernando Valley. Hence, the vests.

As I hopped into the back of the ambulance, I found Crook, a fellow student from Class 36, replacing the batteries in the cardiac monitor. Like me, Crook had been assigned to Station 38, albeit on a different shift with different preceptors. He'd just finished his first twenty-four hours so I was eager for details.

"Just know your shit," he said, looking pale and haggard.

"That's it?" I asked.

"And we're down one backboard," he replied, grabbing his backpack next to the captain's chair. "Good luck out there."

I was disconcerted Crook didn't say more now, but I shook it off and started on my inventory. I began with the Lifepak 15 cardiac monitor. The batteries were fully charged so I tested the defibrillator with a test shock and checked the printer paper. Next, I methodically sorted through each pocket of the carrying case that held the monitor, writing down the contents. Left big pocket: BP cuff; pulse oximetry, and 4-lead ECG cables. Top pocket: adult and child defibrillator pads; safety glasses; large adult BP cuff; pediatric cuff; N95 mask (for tuberculosis patients); and a six-pack of "tender toes," ECG electrodes for pediatric patients.

Just then, a firefighter in workout gear stuck his head in. "Any questions so far?"

I hadn't seen him before. "No, sir."

"I'm Rob," he said, extending a hand and explaining that Eddie was on vacation with his family. "So I'll be your second preceptor today and a few shifts over the course of your internship." Rob had served as a Marine prior to being hired by LAFD and still wore a high and tight haircut.

I thanked him, and he told me to let him know if I needed anything, he'd be on the treadmill in back.

That morning began calmly—I could hear country music playing as Rob hit the treadmill (instead of the rap I'd expected, given L.A.'s illustrious rap history, it turned out that Station 38 favored Go Country, 105.1). Country music was blasting as Captain Turner reviewed the station log, Carlos whipped up some scrambled eggs, and Tim and Nick read the morning paper in the kitchen. And country music was playing as the station lights flickered, tones sounded, and our first call came in: *Engine and rescue . . . unconscious.*

Denise Martin lived with her eighty-five-year-old mother across town on King Street, in a modest beige stucco single-family home with a black Suburban parked under a carport. As we pulled up, I leapt out the back of the ambulance, my heart racing. I was already wearing my exam gloves and safety glasses, like some cartoon character named Ricky Rescue. Tim just shook his head at me.

"When you see your patient, let me know if you think she's critical," Tim said as we pulled out the gurney.

The cardiac monitor, airway bag, and first-in bag full of medications sat atop the gurney, easily accessible. We steered the gurney past a gate and to the front door, flanked by the firefighters from the engine.

"Paramedics!" I announced, knocking three times quickly.

"Hey, guys," Denise Martin, a heavyset woman in her fifties, said matter-of-factly. "Mom's in the living room."

We followed Denise through the kitchen. It smelled of chicken broth and the counters were covered with tortilla strips, cotija cheese, and shredded chicken. She was making tortilla soup.

"Start talking," said Tim, tapping my shoulder. "Let's go."

I asked Denise why she'd called us out today.

"The usual," she replied. "I couldn't wake her."

I saw her mother, Margaret Martin, lying motionless on the couch with one arm hanging limply to the floor.

"Critical," I whispered to Tim as I hurried over to determine responsiveness.

Denise returned to the kitchen and continued stirring the soup. "I'll be in here if you need me."

I couldn't understand her lack of worry.

I tapped Margaret's shoulder. "Hello, ma'am," I said. "Can you open your eyes for us?"

Margaret didn't open her eyes, but, when I squeezed the tip of her finger for a pain response, she moaned slightly.

"I need to hear what you're thinking," Tim said.

"And put the firefighters to work," added Rob. "Let's go, run the call!"

"Airway's patent," I said, before throwing on a stethoscope and listening to lung sounds. "Breathing sounds good."

"What's good?" Tim demanded.

"Normal rate and rhythm with good tidal volume," I replied. "And clear lungs."

"Yes, but she's altered," said Tim. "She should be on the pulse oximetry or oxygen by now."

"Come on! You've got firefighters standing around doing nothing," Rob said, clapping his hands. "Let's go, start delegating."

I asked Bryan to put Margaret on a non-rebreather mask at 15 liters per minute and checked her circulation. Her pulse was strong and regular but her skin was pale, cool, and clammy. I asked Nick to patch her up to the ECG and Carlos to take a set of vitals.

"You haven't stated what the chief complaint is," said Tim, "and I don't know what protocol you're following."

"Chief complaint is altered," I replied.

"She's all patched up," said Nick moments later.

I looked at the monitor—a normal sinus rhythm and good oxygen levels.

"Vitals all within normal limits," said Carlos, removing the stethoscope from his ears.

When Tim asked what could cause someone to be altered, I recalled the mnemonic N.O.T.S.—narcotics; oxygen (lack of); trauma, toxins (overdose), or telemetry (cardiac dysrhythmias); stroke, seizures, sugar (low). "I'd like to get a history on her, but she's altered," I lamented.

"Who could you ask?" Tim said.

Denise was still stirring the soup in the kitchen. "The daughter."

"History of diabetes," Denise told me, "hypertension, and acid reflux."

When I asked if this had happened before, Denise fished out a chicken bone with a fork and said, "All the time. She forgets to take her insulin."

That explains the nonchalant attitude, I thought, hurrying back to the living room, where Tim and Rob waited with a blood sugar reading that was below normal levels.

"Blood sugar should've been one of the first things you checked," Tim said. "Transport or treat on scene?"

"We can fix this," I said. "Start an IV and treat on scene."

I pulled out my IV supplies and placed an IV catheter in Margaret's arm. As I screwed on the saline lock, I asked Bryan to pull out the dextrose. I'd administer this syrup-thick solution to raise her blood sugar and wake her up.

As I gave the dextrose, Margaret woke up almost immediately, blinking her eyes open with a dazed, worried look.

"Hi, Margaret," I said gently. "We're with the fire department. Your blood sugar was low."

Margaret nodded, signaling she understood. Minutes later, when I asked where she was, as well as the date, her birthday, and the name of the President of the United States, she answered all my questions correctly. We took another set of vitals and checked her blood sugar again to make sure it was normal, then disconnected the oxygen.

Margaret didn't want to go to the hospital, so we instructed her daughter to make her a sandwich and had Margaret sign an Against Medical Advice form, acknowledging that we advised her to go to the hospital and that she understood the risks for refusing treatment. Then we picked up our trash from the call—the empty box of dextrose, syringes, catheters, gauze wrappers—and my first run of internship was over.

July

Baptism by Fire

As we drove off, Tim said I'd receive all "1s" (failures to perform) on the call and listed many improvement areas—engage earlier; work faster; delegate tasks to the firefighters on the engine; obtain a medical history from family on scene if the patient is altered; and check blood sugar earlier. "But overall, not a bad run out of the gate," Tim said. "And once you arrived at a treatment plan, you did well."

I was thrilled. Certainly, I had a lot of things to improve on, but I'd nailed the IV on my first attempt and pushed dextrose for the first time, reversing a diabetic coma, and witnessed my patient transition from barely responsive to alert and oriented. *Internship is easy*, I thought, *I'm definitely out in twenty shifts.*

It was 10:15 a.m. now and life returned to normal at Station 38. I restocked the dextrose and IV supplies and oxygen mask. Rob cranked the country music up and hopped back on the treadmill. Captain Turner returned to his office to answer some e-mails. Nick reheated his eggs. Tim found the Sports section of the *L.A. Times,* and I started back on my inventory—*five adult non-rebreather masks, ten adult nasal cannulas, five pediatric non-rebreather masks*—and it was about that time that someone in a gray minivan rolled up beside Diego Ruiz, biking home from the store, and fired four rounds.

"*Rescue only. A shooting . . .*" dispatch announced over the loudspeaker, the electronic voice echoing off the apparatus floor.

I couldn't believe my ears. *Who shoots someone this early in the morning? And why isn't the engine responding with us?*

"The gangsters are up early," Nick said as I squeezed into my ballistic vest and hopped on the ambulance. "Be safe out there!"

We thundered out of the station, took a right on Avalon, a left on the Pacific Coast Highway, and raced to the call.

"Engine 85 from Harbor City will be on scene with us," Tim yelled above the siren roar. "Rescue 85 is on another call, so we're giving them a medical aid."

A GSW, I thought, replaying the steps of running a traumatic full arrest in my mind. *On shift one, my second call!* Did I feel ready? It didn't matter. I knew I had to *be* ready because, as we turned down a side street, I spotted firefighters from Engine 85 treating a nineteen-year-old victim under a tree with a gunshot wound and we were arriving in:

Three seconds.

Two seconds.

One second.

And then the locks of the ambulance popped open and I was pulling out the gurney and steering it around a mangled bicycle and bullet casings and then a police officer was hurrying over to me and saying, "He was biking home from the store when a minivan rolled up, yelled, 'Eastside,' and started firing," and then I could hear the boy's mother and sister crying from their house across the street and then I was at the patient's side and it was go time.

As I set the cardiac monitor down, a paramedic from Engine 85 attempted to give me a report. "Nineteen-year-old male, single bullet wound to his—"

But I blazed right past him and started assessing the teenager, who was still under the tree, wincing in pain. He had a single bullet wound above his right ankle.

"What's your name?" I asked.

"Diego," he replied, gasping.

Diego's head was shaved and he wore a white T-shirt, a black rosary around his neck, sagging jean shorts, and the Wilmington zip code—90744—tattooed on his forearm.

"Where are you right now?"

"In front of my house."

When I asked Diego to tell me what time it was, he got angry. "Man, I just answered all these questions!" he hollered. "My fuckin' leg!"

I quickly checked the gunshot area. A dime-sized entrance wound with no bleeding.

The paramedic from Engine 85 who'd attempted to give me a report grabbed his stethoscope and walked away, leaving me with two firefighters from the engine. One had a cardboard splint and the other held gauze and tape.

"You want us to start splinting?" one asked.

I told them I wanted to check ABCs first. "Airway's patent. Breath sounds clear and equal . . ."

"Are you going to get me out of this mud?" Diego howled, sitting in a sprinkler puddle.

Tim hurried over. "Load him up and let's get him going," he said, clapping his hands.

"Okay to splint?" the firefighter asked again.

"Yeah," I replied, checking Diego's pupils. "Equal and reactive."

The two firefighters quickly wrapped Diego's leg and helped me assist him to the gurney. As we loaded him onto the ambulance, I saw the paramedic from Engine 85 talking to Tim and he appeared agitated. Looking back, that was the first sign I'd botched the call.

"Where to?" Rob yelled from the driver's seat.

I directed him to our closest trauma center—"Harbor-UCLA"—and he punched it.

The second sign I'd botched the call came when Tim radioed the nurse at Harbor-UCLA with a report and I realized my assessment was hurried and I hadn't fully inspected the mechanism that had caused the injury. What kind of gun? What range was he shot at? Was there an exit wound? Any associated trauma with diving off his bike? How was the circulation, motor function, and sensation (CMS) of Diego's leg before we'd splinted? How was CMS after? I had no answers for these important questions. Hoping to redeem myself, I started an IV and gave Diego some morphine for pain.

The third sign I'd botched the call came when we entered the ER at Harbor-UCLA, where I found a trauma team of a half dozen nurses and doctors waiting for a report.

"Start talking," a doctor announced as we entered.

The ER staff at Harbor-UCLA were well versed in treating GSW victims. On some years, it wasn't uncommon for the hospital to see over a hundred patients with bullet wounds during L.A.'s "shooting season" from July through September.

Tim looked over at me. "Go with your report!"

"Nineteen-year-old boy with—"

"Can't hear you!" a nurse interjected.

"Nineteen-year-old boy. Chief complaint leg pain, secondary to being shot," I said, raising my voice. "Patient states—"

"You need to talk *and* move him to the hospital bed," said Tim, grabbing the bedsheet underneath Diego.

I grabbed the edges of the sheet at his head and we lifted him over. As we did, the nurses rushed in, cutting away the gauze and removing the cardboard splint. "His vitals were normal and we started an IV and gave morphine," I said.

"Any exit wounds?" one nurse asked, inspecting the small hole where the bullet entered.

"Nope," I declared.

Just then, the nurse pointed to a hole on the inside of Diego's leg. "I've got an exit wound right here."

Tim took a look then recoiled back to me. "You missed that?"

"I don't know how," I replied. "I'm sorry."

"Did you even look?" asked a nurse.

"I tried."

"No," said Rob, "you raced right by the medic from 85 who was trying to give you a report and loaded him up without checking."

When the doctor quizzed me about every aspect of the shooting—the gun, the distance, the number of shots fired, and the range—I had no solid answers and felt awful.

Did my missing the exit wound compromise Diego's care that day? Thankfully, not in the least. While our treatment and hospital destination wouldn't have changed in this case, such an omission could pose much more serious problems on a future call, and I vowed never to make the same mistake again.

I found Tim and Rob waiting for me out behind the ambulance— the fourth sign. "How do you think that call went?" Tim asked.

"Awful," I replied, shaking my head.

Tim agreed and said I needed to relax on scene. "It's not your emergency," he said. "You being all amped up doesn't help anyone. You have to be the calm amid the chaos."

Next, Rob critiqued the way I'd interacted with the paramedic from Engine 85 during the patient handoff. "He'd performed a full assessment and you blazed right by him," Rob said. "How do you think that makes him feel?"

"Not good," I said.

"And then, the patient got angry because you started repeating all the same questions he'd just been asked."

I apologized. "I assumed you wanted me to perform a full assessment each and every time."

And yet, Tim said, I also needed to perform a better physical assessment. "You shouldn't miss an exit wound," he said. "Get your hands on your patient and assess for everything—CMS, deformity, tenderness."

"Got it," I said, scribbling notes in the pocket-sized notebook I'd decided to carry for such instances.

Rob also told me to cut away the clothes on every GSW victim to search for hidden bullet wounds. "What's the first thing people do when they're shot at?" he asked. "They raise their hands like this," he said, demonstrating. "He could've easily been shot under his armpits."

Tim added, "The hospital is going to cut away their clothes anyway. You're just making their job easier."

Rob said he also put GSW victims on a backboard. "Not so much for spinal precautions, but in order to have a hard surface to perform CPR if they go into traumatic arrest," he explained. "And it's easy to transfer them to the hospital bed."

Lastly, Tim said I need to improve my report to the doctors. "You need to be able to talk and work at the same time," he began, "and for your report, they want a sixty-second rundown on the patient: age, sex, chief complaint, a quick description of the injury, and other findings during your rapid trauma exam."

"Got it," I said, jotting notes.

I hoped Tim and Rob would end with some good points about the call—about my nailing the IV and pushing morphine—but they just told me to load up, and took their seats in the front cab. It was 11:45 a.m. on the first day of my field internship. I'd already started two IVs; pushed two new medications; responded to a shooting;

driven Code 3 to the hospital; pissed off a paramedic from Station
85; and had my butt chewed out by the UCLA trauma team and
Tim and Rob behind the ambulance.

And it wasn't even lunchtime yet.

I finished my inventory in four hours and we ran two more calls
that afternoon—an eighty-five-year-old woman complaining of
general weakness and a seventy-five-year-old man who wasn't acting normal. The calls weren't as critical as our first two but Tim
and Rob still rode me hard—*engage earlier; verbalize your findings;
delegate tasks; work faster!*

Prior to internship, I'd assumed the time in between calls at the
station would be relaxing, but I was quickly learning it was nearly
as stressful as the calls.

"After you," Captain Turner said to me that evening, gesturing
to a stack of plates. It was dinnertime, and we were all in the kitchen.

"Thank you for the offer, sir," I said, stepping aside. "But I'll go
last."

"You should go first," replied Captain Turner. "The rescue will
catch a run before the engine."

Should I go through the dinner line first? If so, would this upset
the chain of command? Or should I refuse, which might be inter-
preted as disobeying a direct order from my captain? I was to have
many uncertain moments like this each and every day of internship.

"I'll go last," I said, standing my ground.

For dinner, Bryan had whipped up a stir-fry of some half-
baked—literally—steak and vegetables in a dark pool of soy sauce.

"This is awful! Tastes like stir-fried beef jerky," said Tim, struggling to chew.

"More like Wilmington dog," joked Nick, his face contorting
from the taste.

"I'm doing jaw-zercise," said Carlos, laughing. "It's so salty, I'm going to need a water pill to make me pee!"

I wanted to laugh along, but didn't know if doing so would lead to my being accepted as one of the guys—or be seen as disrespectful. Was laughing a failure criterion during field internship? And what about the movie *Wedding Crashers*, being shown on the flat-screen TV in the corner—was I allowed to sneak a peek? I decided not to risk it. I quickly finished my meal, hopped on the dishes, then wandered out onto the apparatus floor to wash the ambulance.

The sun had set outside and dusk was settling on the city like a blue hazy carpet. Parents called their children inside, locking the doors after them. On Avalon Boulevard, shop owners pulled down security gates and hurried to their cars, glancing over their shoulders. Streetlights blinked on. A distant siren. Palm tree shadows. I had the sense that everyone was battening down the hatches in preparation for a great storm. And perhaps they were.

Night falling on the City of Angels.

"It can get a little hot when the sun goes down," Tim said, taking down the flag outside the station, and I knew he wasn't talking about weather.

When he finished, Tim hit the button to close the doors on the apparatus floor. They chugged down the track like a train. A part of me didn't want the doors to close because it meant the day was over, but I sure as hell didn't want them to stay open. The doors made a loud, halting sound when they hit the floor and then everything fell silent. Who knew the face of the city I'd see when they opened again?

"Most interns struggle after dark," Tim said, disappearing back into the kitchen.

I stayed up until midnight to ensure I was the "last up to bed" and then climbed the steep stairs leading to the second floor, where a narrow hallway led past the locker room. I showered quickly, my ears attentive in case a call came in, and then changed into shorts and my UCLA T-shirt. I'd left the rest of my equipment beside Rescue 38 so that when the tones sounded, I could just step into my boots, pull up my turnouts, and hop on.

The bunkroom was large. Beds lined all four walls and weight equipment sat at the center. In the dark, the bench press, dumbbells, and multipurpose weight machine looked like prehistoric insects. I'd claimed the bed closest to the door and a small nightstand with a telephone on it. We were dispatched to calls differently at night. Rather than the alarm tones and dispatch coming on the loud-speaker, at night the telephone rang loudly if the rescue ambulance was needed. If the call required the engine, the overhead lights in the bunkroom blazed on. And if both the engine and rescue were needed, the lights and telephone would activate at the same time, waking you out of sleep with a mortarlike barrage.

What discomfort about station life I felt during the day was made up for by the bunkroom at night. It had a Bat Cave darkness and an air-conditioning unit that blew a strong, cold wind, lulling you to sleep instantly with its meditative hum. But around two a.m. all hell broke loose—the lights blazed on, the phone rattled the nightstand with its ring, and I found myself tearing down the stairs to respond to a forty-five-year-old man who was unconscious.

We arrived at a small, dark house on Gulf Avenue with a black tarp substituting for a missing part of the roof.

An elderly woman in a nightgown answered the door. "It's my son," she said, leading us down a boot-wide trail through the living room. They were hoarders, and the rest of the room was an avalanche of clothes, newspapers, magazines, trash, and pizza boxes that rose to knee level.

"What's going on tonight?" I asked, carrying the cardiac monitor and first-in bag.

"I can't wake my son."

"When did this start?"

"Twenty minutes ago."

"What medical problems does he have?"

"Schizophrenia. Depression. And he's bipolar."

We turned down a hallway, lit by a single white bulb hanging down from a water-stained ceiling. We were deep in the house now, but could we get out? The woman stopped and gestured to the bedroom on the right. "Christopher's in there."

"Christopher," I said, kicking my way through the trash to his bedside. "What's going on tonight?"

Christopher weighed four hundred pounds. He lay supine in his bed with his arms extended at his sides, breathing loudly.

"Sir," I said, tapping his shoulder, "can you open your eyes for us?"

Christopher didn't respond. I quickly checked my ABCs—all normal—but when I went to assess his pupils, he clamped his eyelids closed. This told me Christopher wasn't truly unconscious. If he were, he'd lose his eyelash reflex.

"It's the fire department," I said. "We're here to help you." And it was about that time that Christopher began emitting this creepy noise—a guttural growl that rose up from somewhere deep inside him and vibrated the bed with a staccato shake.

"Keep the call moving forward," Tim said from my left. "Let's go. Make decisions."

As Christopher's growling grew louder, I started to panic a bit. *Vital signs!* I thought, *That's something I can check.* I grabbed the BP cuff and, without looking, handed it to the firefighter on my right. "Go ahead and get me a BP," I said. My delegation was good but there was only one problem—I'd handed the blood pressure cuff to Captain Turner, the most senior member of our crew. By the time I realized who had the cuff, it was too late.

The rest of the call would go smoothly. Christopher's vital signs were within normal limits and there was no sign of trauma, seizure, stroke, low blood sugar, or overdose. Then, using the interview tactics of clarification, reflection, repetition, and compassion, I would discover Christopher wasn't altered—he just wasn't taking his medications and had had an argument with his mother. I convinced Christopher to go to the hospital, where I was able to deliver a solid patient report to the nursing staff at the Kaiser Medical Center in Harbor City.

But absolutely none of this would matter, since I'd ordered my captain to get me a blood pressure.

"Sure," Captain Turner had said, wrapping the cuff around Christopher's upper arm, "I can get you a blood pressure . . ."

We didn't get any more calls that night but it didn't matter—I still didn't sleep. And I couldn't help but intuit that I was getting the cold shoulder from the firefighters at Station 38. What else would explain Bryan, Nick, and Carlos leaving at shift change in the morning without saying a word? All Tim said was, "Eddie's back on your next shift. Be ready."

When I gave Crook my morning report, he didn't offer much consolation, either. "You did what?" he exclaimed. "And they didn't fail you on the spot?"

I hoped to catch Captain Turner in his office on my way out to apologize, but, when I knocked, no one answered. Was the office empty? Or did Captain Turner just not want to see me? Either way, I knew I'd dug myself into a hole and would have to shovel myself out on shift two.

"Put people to work," Mrs. Medina had advised. Oh, I had—stupidly, comically, tragically.

I went home and slept for a few hours, then woke up around noon and started prepping for my second shift.

On shift two, I was back again at Station 38, planning to knock on the door at Captain Turner's office. Would he accept my apology? Or would he sign my termination papers?

When I arrived at the station that morning and received my morning report from Crook, he looked more pale and despondent than ever. Crook confessed he was having trouble with his preceptors. "One guy used to be Special Forces or something," he said, "and anytime I ask the other guy a question, he just tells me to look it up."

"Hang in there," I said. "They'll probably ease up."

As Crook left, I started on inventory. Tim and Eddie arrived moments later and grabbed their equipment out of the lockers next to the ambulance.

"How'd he do, Tim?" Eddie asked, as if I wasn't standing two feet away.

"The only thing good about him is his white teeth," Tim replied, tossing his brush coat on the rig.

I assumed Tim was joking, but when he handed me my daily evaluation from my first shift, I found the form filled out entirely with "1s"—*fails to perform*. The only glimmer of hope was in the comments section at the bottom: *Kevin accepted the responsibility of patient care. He seems to have a well-rounded knowledge base.*

As Tim and Eddie went to work out, I finished my inventory and then sought out Captain Turner.

"I wanted to apologize for asking you to get that blood pressure on my last shift," I told him. "I didn't see who was behind me. The patient was growling, and I just panicked."

I was ready for Captain Turner to inform me he'd spoken with Mrs. Medina and that I was being yanked from the field, but he waved the blood pressure incident off as no big deal. I was to learn that Captain Turner was one of those rare breed of men who was as humble as he was accomplished. There were other parts of the call that concerned him more, however, such as how I'd neglected my own safety.

"Anytime you go into a house like that, you need to devise a plan for getting out," he began. "I always make sure I got a clear path to the door and never turn my back on a psych patient because they'll spring on you in an instant."

His biggest concern, though, was with my patient interaction—I was too robotic and mechanical.

"Probably because I'm stressed," I said, nodding.

Captain Turner agreed. "But our job as paramedics and firefighters is to *talk* to people," he said. "Don't think of them as calls—think of them as visits. This person has asked you over to their house for a visit and you're there to see how you can help them."

I thanked Captain Turner for his time and found Tim on the apparatus floor. He handed me a bucket of soapy water and a towel. "We're cleaning floorboards today," he said with great pride. "This is a fire station, not a gas station."

I knelt at the base of the staircase and started scrubbing. Meanwhile, at a duplex on Van Tress Avenue on the west side of Wilmington, Father Shanahan was checking on one of his parishioners. It wasn't like Harold Rosenburg to miss nine o'clock Mass. Moments later, the lights flickered and alarm tones sounded: *Engine and rescue . . . cardiac arrest.*

"First thing to do is get on scene and start good, high-quality CPR," Tim said as we pulled out the gurney beside the two-story apartment complex. Father Shanahan was waiting for us curbside, dressed in black clerical pants and a shirt with a white tab collar. "Harold's in the living room," he said with sad eyes.

I hurried toward the house, my mind running through the different cardiac arrest algorithms for V-tach, V-fib, asystole, and PEA.

Eddie and Tim followed a few steps behind me, pulling on their safety gloves as they walked. Father Shanahan had propped the front door open with a chair so I left the gurney outside. I grabbed the cardiac monitor with my right hand, the first-in bag with my left, and hustled in to find Mr. Rosenburg lying facedown over a coffee table, dead.

Harold Rosenburg was a sixty-six-year-old man, barefoot and dressed in shorts and a white T-shirt. His skin was pale, with dark purple patches visible on the undersides of his arms and legs. He'd fallen face forward onto the knee-high table at the center of the room, his arms and head hanging rigidly over the side. His yellowish eyes were wide open and a string of snot hung from the cavern of his right nostril like a stalactite. I set my equipment down as Eddie, Tim, and the firefighters on the engine entered.

"What are you thinking?" Eddie said, amped up. "Start talking. Start treating."

"Obvious lividity," I replied. "He's probably been down for hours."

"So you're saying he's 814 criteria," asked Tim, "meaning we should withhold resuscitation?"

"Yes, sir."

Eddie reminded me my assessment didn't end there. "Let's go, hurry up!"

I grabbed my stethoscope. "I need to verify there's no respiratory, cardiac, or neuro activity."

"Don't say it—do it," Eddie barked. "Get it done."

Mr. Rosenburg's airway was open, so I placed the stethoscope buds in my ears and listened for lung sounds on his back and looked for any sign of breathing. Nothing. Next, I placed my first two fingers in the crease of his neck below the jaw and checked his carotid pulse for sixty seconds. His neck was swollen and his skin felt refrigerated.

Tim reminded me to verbalize my findings.

"Airway's open and no breathing or pulse," I said, grabbing my penlight and crouching down on the floor to check his pupils. They were wide and unresponsive.

"Pupils fixed and dilated," I said, sitting up. "He meets all of the 814 criteria for determining death in the field."

Father Shanahan peeked in the door.

"I'm sorry, sir," Tim said. "There's nothing we can do."

Father Shanahan nodded. He knew. We gathered up our gear, called the coroner, and locked the door on our way out.

Back at the station, Tim and Eddie said they'd known it would be an 814 the moment we arrived on scene and spotted Father Shanahan standing curbside. "There was no panic or urgency in him," Eddie explained. "Many times, you can tell how critical your patient is by watching how people greet you at the ambulance."

Tim said he wanted me to really process the scene on our next call. "Take a deep breath and do a good scene size-up," he said. "Who's standing outside to greet you? How do they look? Are they panicked? What are they doing?"

"Got it," I said, grabbing my sponge and returning to the floor-boards.

An hour later, we were dispatched to another cardiac arrest. And my scene size-up? A family barbecue. Fifteen people waiting outside. And everyone screaming, shouting, or crying. Absolute chaos.

As I hurried to the front door of the single-family home, I wondered who I should speak with to get information about the patient. The tall, muscular man wearing a blue Dodgers hat, shouting, "Hurry up!"? It couldn't be the little girl standing with a doll, frozen with fear, or the hysterical woman pulling at her hair with tears streaming down her cheeks.

Just then, another woman, this one with shoulder-length brown hair and wearing glasses, appeared at the front door. "I'm Candice," she said, grabbing my arm and leading me into the living room. "It's my mom. She's in the back."

Candice gave me a quick rundown on her mom. Fifty-six years old. Stage 4 cancer. Found ten minutes before. No CPR prior to our arrival.

As we arrived at a bedroom, Candice stepped aside. "Please, help her," she said, her voice quivering.

"We'll do everything we can," I said, hurrying in.

Davita Rodgers had collapsed in a small bedroom with patterned wallpaper. She was faceup on the floor, wedged between two twin beds. Cancer had clearly ravaged her body; you could see the outline of her bones under her skin. I immediately knelt and checked her carotid pulse. Absent. There wasn't space to work her up in the tiny bedroom but I also didn't want to delay CPR any longer, so I placed my two hands on her lower breastbone and started compressions until the rest of the crew arrived. "One and two and three and four . . ." I said, as her thoracic cavity recoiled up and down with the force.

Eddie hurried in after me. "Get her in the living room," he said. "Now!"

Bryan lifted the woman's legs. I grabbed under her arms and we carried her out of the bedroom. The woman was light and her arms hung rigidly at her sides. *That's strange,* I thought. We raced up the hall into the living room, where Nick and Carlos had moved aside a sofa chair and a toy train set, and Captain Turner had cleared out the family.

We set the woman down and I immediately instructed Bryan and Carlos to drop an oropharyngeal airway and begin CPR at a rate of thirty compressions to two breaths with bag-valve mask attached to high-flow oxygen. Next I pulled out defibrillation pads and stuck them on Ms. Rodgers's right upper chest and left flank. After two minutes of CPR, I told Bryan and Carlos to stop CPR while I checked for a pulse and the ECG rhythm.

"Asystole," I said, verifying the flatline on another lead. "Continue CPR . . ."

As they hopped back on compressions, Eddie and Tim asked me if I'd noticed anything unusual about the woman when I'd carried her.

"No," I said, yanking out my IV equipment from the first-in bag.

Tim asked if I'd seen her arms when we'd carried her. "They were rigid," he said. "She's got rigor."

I told Tim I had noticed that, but the family said she'd only been down ten minutes.

Eddie checked Ms. Rodgers's jaw. Rigid and stiff. "The family may have just found her, but she passed a few hours ago," he said.

"Want me to continue compressions?" asked Bryan.

Eddie and Tim looked over at me. "He's the lead medic."

I instructed Bryan and Nick to stop and confirmed there was no respiratory, cardiac, or neurological activity in the same way I had on the previous call. "She meets 814 criteria," I said, standing. "We have to tell the family."

Eddie corrected me. "You have to tell them."

Captain Turner opened the front door and the family filed in slowly. Their eyes darted from us to the body and then back to us. When Candice appeared in the doorway, I started speaking. "I'm sorry to inform you but your mother has passed away," I said. "There's nothing we can do . . ."

Elisabeth Kübler-Ross, the late Swiss American psychiatrist, described five stages of dealing with grief and here came the first—denial.

"She can't be gone," Candice said, eyes welling with tears. "No . . ."

The second stage of grief was anger. "You're not going to try to save her?" the man in the blue Dodgers hat bellowed, pushing his way to the front of the crowd. "Do something!"

We'd seen a woman beyond resuscitation, but what the family saw was a group of paramedics and firefighters who'd spent a mere two minutes trying to save the woman's life. Captain Turner recognized this immediately. He explained our reasoning to the family in more detail and then took the man in the Dodgers hat outside to talk in private.

"Maybe if we'd found her sooner," said the woman who was still pulling at her hair and crying. "If only we'd called quicker . . ." Here was the third stage of grief—bargaining.

Just then, the girl with the doll appeared in the doorway and burst into tears. This was the fourth stage—depression. "I miss Grandma," she wailed. "Why did Grandma have to die?"

"Somebody take her out!" said Candice.

The girl's mother led her outside, leaving a tear trail.

When she was gone, Candice knelt down on the living room floor next to her mother. Kissed her on her forehead and fixed the part in her hair. "She's in a better place now," Candice said, slowly moving into the fifth stage—acceptance. "I'm sure you're looking down on us from heaven right now, Momma," she said, delivering another kiss.

We gathered our equipment, so the family could have their privacy, and on my way out, I apologized to Candice and the man in the Dodgers hat for their loss. "Thank you for your help," he said, shaking my hand. "I'm sorry I got a little heated."

As we waited in the ambulance for the police or coroner to arrive (either of whom could issue a death certificate and order removal of the body), I asked Eddie how to tell who the best person to talk to was about patient information in a crowded scene.

"Find the person who comes out to meet you and looks you in the eyes," he advised. "That's the one."

A half hour later, an LAPD officer arrived and we turned the scene over to him. As we drove off, Tim said that as paramedics we couldn't always change the outcome of a call. "But that doesn't mean we can't provide great service," he added, glancing in the rearview mirror as he drove. "We can leave the family saying, 'Those firefighters and paramedics from LAFD were so nice, compassionate, and professional. They made the worst day of my life just a little bit easier.'"

July

All Eyes on Me

My third shift was slow, with just three EMT-level calls—a drunk guy without a medical complaint in an alley, surrounded by empty bottles; a woman having an anxiety attack in front of her family; and a woman complaining of a urinary tract infection. Despite this, Tim's and Eddie's constant nitpicking continued: engage quicker; work faster; don't be so mechanical; work the patient up on scene; work the patient up en route—for being two preceptors on the same shift and from the same department, they had vastly different styles.

Tim wanted me to vocalize everything on scene. "If you don't say something, we don't document it," he said, "and if it's not documented, then we didn't do it." Eddie, on the other hand, wanted me to verbalize only the abnormal findings. "If you're called to fix the faucet, you don't walk into a bathroom and say, 'The door handle works. The light works,'" he said. "No! You only say, 'The left handle of the faucet is leaking.'"

Whose advice to follow? And would swaying to one side or the other alienate my other preceptor?

I'd expected the twenty-four-hour shifts to be exhausting, but I hadn't planned on station life and being around the crew to be so stressful. I walked around in a constant state of anxiety, leaping at the slightest sounds, like the phone ringing or the dryer buzzer.

I also found the calls far different during internship from how they'd been in class. In paramedic school, your patient had only one chief complaint—it was always critical—and always collapsed in the middle of a well-lit room. In the field, however, there was always an obstacle: flights of stairs, broken lights, cluttered apartments. Or else the patient had twenty chief complaints. Or the patient was critical but didn't want to go to the hospital. Despite the stress, however, I was learning a lot and felt so grateful for the opportunity. While I'd only received "1s"—*fails to perform*—on all my runs so far, Tim and Eddie continued to scribble positive comments at the bottom of my daily evaluations: *Kevin fits in well at Fire Station 38 . . . No red flags at this point . . . Learning well and performing at the expected level.*

Unfortunately, I heard that Crook's preceptors weren't saying the same things about him. According to Tim, his preceptors asked what the function of the pancreas was and Crook said he'd have to get back to them. "It produces insulin," Tim said. "It doesn't produce brain. If you don't know that, don't you think you'd know this isn't the right profession for you?" Crook had also dropped the oxygen bottle by accident and broke the regulator, which controls the flow of oxygen from the tank to the patient, then told an oncoming crew the ambulance was down a box of dextrose instead of replacing it himself—a big "no-no."

At that point, I wasn't sure Crook would pass internship. All his confidence was gone. He looked broken. It didn't seem like he'd followed the maxim of "Control what you can control"—he should've known what the pancreas does and replaced the dextrose himself (instead of asking the oncoming crew to do it). All of us struggled—every paramedic intern is an underdog, and I sensed there was a very thin dam holding back a reservoir of doubt about my competency as a paramedic—but making mistakes on scene *and* not having the book knowledge was the kind of one-two punch that sends an intern staggering for failure.

But Crook's biggest mistake was missing a call just after midnight on July 21. Two kids, an eighteen-year-old boy and thirteen-year-old girl, had been shot leaving a recreation center, where ironically they—along with dozens of other kids—had been for the "Summer Night Lights" project, an anti-gang initiative that keeps the parks and rec centers across L.A. open late to keep kids off the streets and reduce violence. As the kids were leaving that night, someone fired into the crowd, wounding the two teens. Engine 38 responded. Rescue 38 pulled out immediately after . . . while Crook was still singing in the shower.

At 11:15 on the morning of my fourth shift, I stood in front of the firefighters at Fire Station 38 giving a proficiency drill on ambulance inventory, and I had one question burning in my mind: *What the hell is a V-Vac?*

The morning had started great. I'd run two calls—one for abdominal pain, the other for back pain—and I'd scored my first "2s" of internship. I'd never been so happy to be labeled "borderline, inconsistent" in my life! When we returned to the station, I'd proactively asked if I could do a proficiency drill on the inventory and now, an hour later, I stood in front of the crew fielding questions like hard-hit grounders.

"What's in the top cabinet to the right of the captain's chair?" Tim asked early in my drill.

"Adult and pediatric masks," I replied. "Pediatric electrodes, an extra roll of printer paper for the cardiac monitor, extra adult and pediatric defibrillation pads, and an end-tidal CO_2 detector for use after intubation."

"What's on the second shelf of the medication cabinet?" Rob asked like a drill sergeant, filling in for Eddie once again.

"Preloads of Narcan, adenosine, and amiodarone," I said. "Two nasal atomizers to spray medication up a patient's nostrils. One 5ml syringe and one 1ml syringe."

When Captain Turner asked about the cabinet above the back doors of the ambulance, I told him: seven rolls of gauze, three trauma dressings, four bottles of normal saline, three sets of soft restraints, and two spit hoods. And that was how it went for the next twenty minutes. They'd name a cabinet and I'd tell them everything in it; or vice versa, I'd tell them where to find a particular piece of equipment.

I was nailing everything . . . until Tim asked about the V-Vac. My mind searched for an answer. Did it refer to a piece of equipment that went by another name? If so, which one?

"To be very honest, sir," I began, "I don't know what that is."

Tim and Rob exchanged looks silently. But I heard an unmistakable sound—the sound of a crack in the dam holding back the reservoir of doubt.

"You don't know?" Tim clarified.

"No, sir," I said again.

Tim informed me a V-Vac was another name for a hand-powered suction device that LAFD used to clear blood and vomit from a patient's airway.

"Thank you," I said, swallowing my impulse to tell him that I'd known it by another name. "I will never forget that."

When Rob asked if there was anything else in the ambulance I didn't know about, I told him no, I knew everything.

He smiled. "Everything?"

"Everything," I said confidently.

"What's in the glove compartment?" Tim asked.

I had never even thought to look in the glove compartment. Was there one? My head dropped with shame.

A tense silence ensued. Now there was water dripping through the crack.

"Know your apparatus," Tim suggested. "Dismissed."

I thanked them for their attention. Moments later came the call: *Engine and rescue . . . chest pain.*

"Here's your chance to redeem yourself," said Tim as we hurried to the rig.

Carol Dwyer had found her husband, Dan, in the laundry room, hunched over the washer, gasping for breath and sweating. After she called 911, Carol had helped her husband sit on the bed they'd shared for the last twenty years, and then hurried outside to wait for help to arrive. At first there was only the hot, So Cal sun but then in the distance she heard the unmistakable whine of sirens approaching. Moments later, Engine 38 sped around the corner, trailed by Rescue 38. Carol hurried to the curb and when the back door of the ambulance opened, she immediately started talking.

"I called for my husband, Dan," she said worriedly. "He's in the bedroom."

"What's going on with him today?" I asked, pulling out the gurney.

"His chest hurts and he's having trouble breathing," Carol said, leading me inside.

The Dwyers lived in a two-story home on Eudora Avenue with a well-manicured lawn and a basketball hoop at the end of a newly paved driveway.

When I asked what kind of medical problems he had, Carol told me that he had high blood pressure, high cholesterol, and diabetes, but no allergies.

We raced into the living room, where a family picture hung above the fireplace. The Dwyers and their two daughters had taken it at the beach, and there was Dan in blue jeans, a white sweater, and a smile that beamed with pride.

Carol led me into their bedroom, where Dan was now seated on the edge of the bed, sweating profusely, in severe respiratory distress.

"What's going on today, sir?" I asked.

"I . . . can't . . . catch . . . my . . . breath," he said, speaking in strained, one-word exertions.

"Do you have any pain?"

"My . . . chest," he managed.

I told Bryan to put Dan on a non-rebreather oxygen mask at 15 liters per minute. Asked Nick to grab me a set of vitals and threw on my stethoscope to listen to breath sounds.

"Respirations rapid and shallow," I said, setting my stethoscope aside and assessing his radial pulse and skin signs. "Weak and rapid," I said to Captain Turner, who was taking notes. "Skin's pale, cool, and moist."

"O_2 is on," said Bryan. "What else you need?"

"Let's get a 12-lead," I said, as Tim handed me four 81mg tablets of aspirin.

It was no longer "wait for the paramedic intern to run the call"—it was "all hands on deck to save this man's life." All signs pointed to a heart attack. I lifted the non-rebreather mask away from Dan's mouth and placed the white tablets on his tongue. "Chew these up and swallow them," I instructed. "It will help your body absorb them faster."

"His blood pressure is tanking," Nick said as he finished taking vitals.

"You want nitro?" Tim asked.

"Not with a BP below 100," I replied.

"I can't get these electrodes to stick," Bryan said. "He's sweating too much."

"Here!" said Carol, tossing us a towel.

As I wiped Dan's chest off, Tim and Rob slapped on electrodes to obtain a 12-lead ECG of his heart.

"Hold still for a moment," I said to Dan, hitting the "acquire" button on the cardiac monitor. I waited for the monitor to capture the rhythm and then, as it started printing, asked Bryan, Carlos, and Nick to load Dan onto the gurney. When the ECG strip finished printing, I tore it off the monitor and saw the ominous "tombstone" morphology in multiple leads with the following interpretation:

Acute MI Suspected

"Let's get going to the hospital," I said, handing the rhythm strip to Tim.

Carol Dwyer kissed her husband good-bye as we wheeled him out and she called after him, "I'll meet you at the hospital!"

Torrance Memorial Hospital was our closest cardiac facility and by the time Tim radioed in with a report, I'd already started an IV and tried to raise Dan's blood pressure with normal saline. No luck. His BP was still tanking, which led me to believe it wasn't a fluid problem. If it was, his heart rate would've been skyrocketing to compensate, but it was still within normal limits. He also wasn't on any beta-blockers, which might've prevented the rapid pulse normally seen in compensating shock. Since it wasn't a volume problem, we needed to "squeeze the container," i.e., find a medication that would constrict the vessels and put the proverbial finger over the hose in order to increase the force of the flow. That left us with one option.

"Dopamine," I said to Tim.

"Good call," Tim replied. "Get it done."

I pulled out the dopamine and drew it up into a 5ml syringe. Then I grabbed a 500ml bag of normal saline. Injected the dopamine and labeled it with a black Sharpie marker. Next, I spiked the bag using a 60 drops/ml drip set and hung it above our primary IV.

"ETA six minutes," Rob yelled from the driver's seat.

I quickly set up the flow rate on the dopamine in accordance with L.A. County policies—one drop every two seconds—and returned to Dan. "How's your chest pain now?" I asked.

"Better," he managed, nodding. "Thank you."

He looked better, too. The sweat on his brow had dried and he was breathing easier. As Rob backed us into the ER bay at Torrance Memorial, I recycled the blood pressure and acquired another 12-lead. Both showed improvement.

"Couple bumps on the way out," I told Dan as we unloaded the gurney and wheeled him into the ER, where a team of doctors once again waited. Unlike on my first shift, I expected the doctors this time. "Fifty-eight-year-old male, chief complaint shortness of breath with chest pain," I said as we transferred Dan to the hospital bed. "Patient states the shortness of breath was unprovoked and came on suddenly when he was doing his laundry."

As the doctors rushed in, I stepped back and continued talking. "We put him on high-flow oxygen, gave him aspirin, started a line, and administered dopamine," I said with a new confidence. "Patient now states he's feeling much better."

When I finished, the nurse signed our electronic patient care report and congratulated me on a job well done. "Strong work!"

Tim and Rob went to grab a soda in the ER staff lounge. "Start cleaning the gurney and we'll meet you at the rig," Tim said, tossing me the keys—clearly a good sign.

As I walked to the ambulance, I was ecstatic. Not only had I stabilized a critical patient in the throes of cardiogenic shock and a massive heart attack, but I'd also gotten him off to the hospital quickly, nailed the IV, and hung dopamine! I couldn't wait to text my classmates and tell them.

When I opened the back door of the ambulance, I discovered the floor littered with trash—alcohol prep pads, 4x4 gauze squares, catheter casings, plastic wrappers from the oxygen mask, bag of normal saline, and the IV drip set, along with the empty vial of dopamine. Due to the critical nature of the call, I hadn't had time to throw anything away. But all this "trash" had been used in the service of saving a life. It was a beautiful mess.

Tim and Rob arrived a few minutes later. By then, I had the gurney dressed and the ambulance sparkling—ready for the next call. I expected to see them celebrating our field save, but they walked in silence.

"What's up?" I asked, sitting on the bench seat.

Tim told me Dan had gone into cardiac arrest. "He was chatting with the doctors and then he said the pain in his chest was getting worse, and he coded."

When I waved this off as intern hazing, Tim told me I could go have a look. "They're doing CPR right now," he said sadly.

Suddenly I realized they weren't joking.

"You probably spoke some of the last words he ever heard," Tim said as we pulled out.

We ran another call later that night for a thirty-four-year-old white guy with a history of drug abuse who was altered. He lived with his mother in a weekly motel on the Pacific Coast Highway next to a liquor store, and when I asked his mom if there was a chance he was on methamphetamine she said, "No, 'cause I ain't buying it for him no more . . ."

His mom sat on a rickety chair in baggy sweatpants, holding a cigarette in her bony fingers. Her son sat on the edge of a single mattress on the floor. The mattress had no sheets but did have food stains. The woman and her son were the Madonna and bambino of meth. Weeping sores covered both their faces. Meth causes tactile hallucinations, which often makes users think bugs are crawling under their skin, so they scratch and scratch until the bugs disappear . . . but then so does the high, so out comes the lighter and glass pipe once again. We ended up taking the son to Kaiser

Medical Center in Harbor City, but not before I knelt on the carpet, which was wet and ripe with urine—lesson learned.

I showered back at the station and crawled into bed, anticipating a sweet, sound sleep. But as soon as I shut my eyes, images from the heart attack call returned. The family photo . . . the ECG readout—***Acute MI Suspected*** . . . the scared look on Dan's face as he struggled to breathe. Had the hospital been able to save him? Lying there, I replayed every moment of the call in my mind. Could I have done more? Worked faster? Been more encouraging?

I knew I'd done everything I could've, but that did little to quiet the questions. "You probably spoke some of the last words he ever heard," Tim had said. What were those words—"a couple bumps on the way out"—as I unloaded the gurney? As the night wore on, I was desperate for answers, but the bunkroom was pitch-black and all I heard was the roar of the air-conditioning unit. It made me shiver.

At six the following morning, I met Crook at the rescue and gave him my off-going report. "The rig is stocked," I said, grabbing my ballistic vest from the captain's chair. "We used a vial of dopamine and gave an albuterol treatment but I replaced those."

"Got it," he said, grabbing the monitor to replace the batteries.

"Have a great shift!"

"I'll try," he said, starting his inventory.

That was the last time I ever saw Crook. When I returned for duty on my next shift, he was nowhere to be found and his preceptors gave me my morning report. They didn't tell me where Crook went and I didn't ask. As they handed me the keys to Rescue 38 and my first month of internship came to an end, I felt the heat turn up and stakes rise exponentially. Crook was gone and, now, all eyes at Station 38 were on one intern.

Me.

August

A Black Cloud

As August began, Tim walked into the laundry room on my seventh shift to give me my first major evaluation. I was busy studying at a little desk they'd set aside for me in the corner.

"You ready for this?" he asked, taking a seat atop the dryer.

"Yes, sir," I said, closing a chapter on abdominal injuries in *Emergency Care in the Streets*.

Eddie had left for another week-long family vacation, but prior to his departure, I'd worked the last two shifts of July with him and he'd grown increasingly disappointed with my performance. According to him, I wasn't being thorough enough. "If you're calling this a panic attack, you need to prove it by showing us everything that it isn't," he said, after we'd responded to a thirty-four-year-old woman who was having difficulty breathing. That meant my doing a full workup and assessing her for a heart attack, congestive heart failure, pneumothorax, pneumonia, pulmonary embolism, and any trauma. "Only after you've ruled out all those can you call it a panic attack!"

He got on me during other calls for not placing a patient in spinal precautions fast enough, for not differentiating between chest pain that was cardiac in nature and pain that was pleuritic (in the lungs), and for asking a patient who was altered about the onset. "No one with an altered level of consciousness knows when it started," he howled. "They're altered!"

At the end of the shift, Eddie told me he expected a huge improvement by the time he got back from his annual family vacation. "We're only hard on you because we care," he said. "This isn't just a paycheck for us."

Now, as Tim gave my first major evaluation, he began, "If this was your twentieth shift, you wouldn't pass."

That wasn't the optimistic opening I'd hoped for.

"But this isn't your twentieth shift," he continued. "It's your seventh shift and seven shifts from now you'll be twice as good as you are today, and three times as competent by your twentieth shift."

Tim outlined my good points—that I showed up on time, well rested, and well prepared, and that I'd accepted the responsibility of patient care. As Tim handed me my written evaluation, I was happy to see that I'd received a "3" (competent) in a number of areas—equipment, medication knowledge, splinting, bleeding control, 12-lead ECG interpretation, and professionalism.

"We can tell you don't have a ton of ambulance experience," he said, "but when we tell you something, we see the change immediately on the next call and we like that."

But I also had some major problem areas—scene management, leading the crew, and my communication with patients. "You're still going off of note cards in your head instead of talking to patients," Tim said. "These are people, not chief complaints."

"I can feel myself being mechanical," I confessed. "I'm hoping this will diminish as I get more comfortable on scene."

"Just remember, it's not your emergency."

Before he left, Tim told me they didn't see a need to extend me beyond twenty shifts at that point. "But watch out, because I think Eddie has it out for you."

As Tim left, I reviewed my major evaluation in more detail. There were a few categories he hadn't filled out—defibrillation; end-tidal capnography, and advanced airway maneuvers like intubation—since I hadn't had the chance to perform these skills yet. But I would soon enough.

Two shifts later, we were dispatched to a private residence, where I found a sixty-six-year-old man lying on the dining room floor. He wasn't breathing and he had no pulse, but no signs of rigor mortis or lividity or any of the other Policy 814 criteria for withholding resuscitation. "Hang in there, Dad!" his son pleaded as we walked in. I told Bryan and Carlos to start CPR and pulled out my defibrillation pads.

It was a cardiac arrest—the real deal.

Our patient, Sebastián Torres, had a history of high blood pressure, renal failure, and diabetes, which had left him with both legs amputated below the knee. He'd been eating dinner with his son, Tomás, when his eyes rolled in the back of his head, the fork dropped from his hand, and he fell lifeless to the floor. Tomás had called 911 and then dragged his dad out from under the table, before standing far away, emotionally overwhelmed.

"Stop CPR and let me check the rhythm on the monitor," I said to Bryan and Carlos after two minutes of chest compressions. "He's in pulseless electrical activity," I said. "Continue CPR. Let's push a round of epinephrine and preoxygenate him for intubation."

We ran the critical calls like a Nascar pit crew—divide and conquer—only instead of four tires, we rushed in to start CPR, control the airway, attach the defibrillation pads, and start an IV. When we walked in, Bryan and Carlos had jumped on chest compressions, Nick had dropped an oropharyngeal airway (OPA) in

Mr. Torres's mouth and began ventilating with a bag-valve mask, I'd patched him to the cardiac monitor, Rob had started an IV, and Captain Turner had begun documenting the call and getting a patient history from Tomás. Once those tasks were completed, I grabbed my laryngoscope handle, a Macintosh blade, and endotracheal tube and lay down on my stomach to attempt my first intubation in the field.

"Thirty seconds of preoxygenation done," said Nick.

I placed a towel under Mr. Torres's head to put it in the sniffing position and then told Nick to stop ventilating and remove the OPA.

As he did, I propped myself up on my elbows. Opened Mr. Torres's mouth with my right hand and, using my left, inserted the laryngoscope at the far right corner of his mouth. I gathered up his tongue slowly in my blade and swept it to the left.

"Twenty-five seconds," said Nick.

Summoning all my strength, I lifted up on his lower jaw at a forty-five-degree angle. Mr. Torres's head was big and heavy so I inched forward on my elbows to get more leverage and lifted higher.

Tim asked if I saw the vocal cords.

"Still looking," I said, peering closer. With his thick neck, Mr. Torres was likely a Mallampati Class 3.

"Twenty seconds," said Nick.

I located the vallecula, the depression just behind the base of the tongue. Inserted my blade and lifted up. As I did, the epiglottis lifted like a trapdoor and I spotted the posterior cartilages of the vocal cords. "Almost there," I replied, my voice trailing off with concentration. I lifted higher and the bottom of the glottic opening appeared. But where were the vocal cords?

"Fifteen seconds."

"Getting low on time," Tim said.

I lifted higher but I still couldn't see the vocal cords. Just then, I remembered the advice from Dr. Sebold, the anesthesiologist I trained with in the operating room, to change something if my intubation attempt wasn't working.

I glanced up to Nick. "Can I get cric pressure, please?"

As he pushed down on Mr. Torres's cricoid cartilage, the notch just below the thyroid cartilage (i.e., Adam's apple), the vocal cords appeared, white and shiny with saliva. "Tube, please!" I said. Rob handed me the ET tube and Bryan paused chest compressions for a moment, as I placed the tube through the vocal cords with great satisfaction.

Next, I quickly inflated the balloon and confirmed placement. "No epigastric sounds and good lung sounds bilaterally," I announced, listening with my stethoscope. Next, we inserted a bite block to secure the tube and added an end-tidal capnography device, which helped us confirm tube placement in the trachea and that our rate of delivering breaths was correct.

By then, two minutes of CPR was up. "Stop compression," I said, jumping to my knees and checking the monitor. "He's still in pulseless electrical activity," I said. "Let's push another round of epinephrine and get going to the hospital."

En route to St. Mary Medical Center in Long Beach, we continued with CPR and administering epinephrine and tried to find the underlying cause of the arrest: was it low blood sugar; dehydration; drug overdose; a missed dialysis treatment?

As we arrived at St. Mary's, the doctors were waiting in the ambulance bay and they hurried alongside us as we wheeled in Mr. Torres. The patient handoff at the hospital was always a relay race, a body substituted for a baton. As we moved Mr. Torres to the bed, I gave my report and then doctors and nurses quickly rushed in.

"I've got a pulse," the nurse immediately announced, checking Mr. Torres's carotid artery.

The pulse appeared as tiny blips of organized electrical activity on the hospital's cardiac monitor.

"Your first field save!" said the nurse, slapping me on my sweat-drenched back.

"Thanks," I replied, softly.

I probably should've been happier. After all, not only was it my first field intubation, my efforts had directly restored a patient's pulse. So why wasn't I? Sure, it had felt great to watch the ET tube pass through the vocal cords and know I had successfully secured the airway, but that call drove home that it didn't matter what we did to a patient—the important thing was the outcome. Yes, our efforts had restored Mr. Torres's pulse, but would any neurological function return? Would he ever finish that meal with his son? Sadly, the answer was mostly likely no.

With a cardiac arrest, survivability drops 10 percent for every minute CPR is withheld. Mr. Torres had been in full arrest for over ten minutes without any CPR being performed prior to our arrival, which meant, statistically, he had little chance at a positive out-come. As we cleared from the hospital that night, I wondered why his son hadn't started CPR. Surely he'd seen it performed in the movies . . . but chances were he'd felt helpless witnessing a cardiac arrest. If so, he wasn't alone. I wondered how many lives could be saved if more people learned hands-only CPR.

I sat down with Tim and Rob in the kitchen to review the run.

"Nice job," Tim began. "We're giving you a '3' on assessment and treatment."

I was thrilled—not only were they the first "3s" I'd scored in major categories during internship, but I'd scored them on a cardiac arrest, often considered one of the most stressful calls we run. But Rob had one main improvement area:

"Your body substance isolation was lacking," he explained. "Your patient had just eaten a full meal and you were a few inches above his mouth intubating him. He could've easily vomited while you were hovering with your tongue wagging out like Michael Jordan."

"Wear a surgical mask next time," Tim added.

We shared a good laugh, and as the rest of the guys filed in for dinner, they all congratulated me on a job well done.

"I couldn't have done it without my team," I said. "Thank you for all your help."

Oops.

"Oh, we're *your* team now?" said Nick.

"Someone's getting a little cocky," joked Captain Turner.

"This intern thinks he walks on water," added Nick.

I tried to apologize, but of course they wouldn't let me get another word in edgewise and the ribbing continued. I played along, knowing that these jokes—as much as earning a "3" on a call—were a sign that I was being accepted at Station 38.

Later, as I wrung out my sponges on the outside patio after washing the ambulance, I felt truly happy. For the first time during internship, I didn't feel an oppressive weight bearing down on my shoulders. I felt like I was finally getting this paramedic puzzle and putting all the pieces together. I tossed my sponge in a bucket and looked up into the sky. I expected a star-filled sky to accompany such an exulted feeling but low fog had blown in and a terrible sense of foreboding seized me. Was it the marine layer, blowing in from the harbor? Or maybe smoke from one of Wilmington's oil refineries? Los Angeles was well-known to have the worst air quality in the United States, and Wilmington, with its refineries and hundreds of diesel trucks traveling from the harbor each day, had arguably the worst air in L.A.

Whatever the fog was that night, I was certain of one thing—it wasn't a white cloud.

A black cloud hovering above Wilmington.

That was the unnerving feeling I had during my next few shifts. But when had it arrived? Was it on shift eight, when we were called to an apartment complex on Cruces Street in Ghost Town for a woman having chest pain, but who whispered to me that her chest didn't hurt? "I'm just scared because my husband is coming home and I'm afraid of what he might do to me and my daughter."

"Where is he?" I asked.

"He's in big boy time-out," the woman's seven-year-old daughter exclaimed happily. And when I asked the woman what "big boy time-out" was, she mouthed "jail."

A black cloud was there when LAFD Rescue 85 out of Harbor City was dispatched for a dead baby and requested a medical aid from us because the twenty-three-year-old mother had overdosed on ecstasy and meth . . . but arrived to find her picking at meth mites under her skin with one hand and holding her six-month-old baby boy, alive and well, in the other. She was so high—twitching and tweaking—she'd mistakenly thought her son was dead. The paramedics from Harbor City ended up transporting the baby to Kaiser Medical Center and we took Mom there a few minutes later.

"I want to see my baby," she whined en route.

I exchanged a look with the police officer riding in the back with me. We weren't swayed by those tattoo tears below her right eye.

"Please, sir," she moaned, "I want to see my baby . . ."

You should've thought about that before you did meth, I thought.

A black cloud was hovering above a private residence where we found an overweight man sitting in the bathtub in a pool of thick, clotted blood. A varicose vein had burst in his leg. When I asked what medical problems he had, he screamed, "Just look at me!"

A black cloud followed me when I walked into an apartment

on McFarland Avenue and a woman opened the door and yelled, *"Socorro! Está muriendo!"* I said, "What?" and she screamed, *"No está respirando!"* and I yelled, "I don't understand!" and she pleaded, *"Por favor!"* and Tim yelled, "Find your patient!" and I hollered, "Where?" and the woman rushed me into the back bedroom where a twenty-three-year-old woman with a congenital birth disease was pale and cyanotic and I squeezed her shoulder and said, "Ma'am, open your eyes!" and she didn't respond so I checked her pulse and then told Bryan to start CPR.

It was still hovering overhead on my eleventh shift, in a different manifestation:

"You need to attack the chief complaint when you arrive on scene!" Eddie screamed at me. *"Immediately!"*

Eddie was back from vacation and I'd never seen him so angry. We were in the ambulance bay at Harbor-UCLA, having just dropped off a fifty-six-year-old woman with symptoms of pneumonia. A half hour earlier, I'd walked into her living room and she'd told me she had chest tightness so I—trying to be more natural and "talk to people" as Tim and Captain Turner had suggested— sat down and started asking my patient history questions about how she'd describe the tightness; when it started; if the tightness moved, and if she had a productive cough. Evidently that wasn't the right thing to do.

"Is checking a patient's vital signs going to save her life?" Eddie hollered. *"Is obtaining a history going to save her life?"*

"No, sir!" I said.

"Correct!" he yelled, as people stopped to watch. *"The only thing that's going to save her life is checking her ABCs and attacking the chief complaint with your interventions!"*

"I agree, sir," I said.

Eddie walked away, then turned around and added that I also needed to speed up on scene.

"You're like molasses!" he shouted. "You're like molasses trying to sink into a sponge!"

I promised him I'd do my best.

"I don't know what was going on when I was away," Eddie said, as veins popped up out of his forehead, "but this can't continue!"

Eddie stormed off, leaving me alone with Tim to dress the gurney.

"My preceptors tried to fail me, too," Tim said, as we buckled up the seat belts, "but I told them that wasn't an option and got my act together."

I loaded up the gurney and we cleared from the hospital. But we hadn't driven a half mile before Eddie looked in the rearview mirror. "Did you replace all the equipment from the last call?" he asked.

"Yes, sir."

Eddie asked if we had the oxygen bottle back in the green airway bag.

"The airway bag is right here on the gurney."

As opposed to most gurneys, the model LAFD used didn't have a place to hang an oxygen bottle. If we used oxygen—as we had on the woman with pneumonia—we placed the bottle in between the patient's ankles at the foot of the gurney. We'd then set the oxygen bottle aside at the hospital when we transferred the patient to a bed in the ER and pick it up before we left. That day, after we'd transferred the woman to the bed, I'd given the doctor a report and turned to find the gurney gone. Naturally I assumed Tim and Eddie had picked up the oxygen bottle, but, when I checked the airway bag, I discovered it empty.

"Do we have all of our equipment?" Eddie demanded again.

"No, sir," I said, "the oxygen bottle is missing."

Eddie slammed on the brakes and turned around. *"That's just crap!"*

I was in internship hell. Forget about a crack in the dam holding back the reservoir of doubt, this was a full flood.

We retrieved the oxygen bottle from the hospital and returned to Station 38. Dinner was a silent, awkward affair. *Not a good day,* Tim would write at the bottom of my daily evaluation. *Still struggling with communication, leadership, and scene management.*

But at 4:17 the following morning, the lights in Fire Station 38 would flash on, the phone would ring, and I'd get my shot at redemption. On Ravenna Avenue, Mia Walker was having contractions that were increasing in frequency and duration. Her water had broken. She had the urge to bear down and all signs pointed to imminent delivery.

As I wiped sleep from my eyes and we raced toward the Walkers' modest two-bedroom home, I sensed this call was not only a chance to deliver a baby but also a chance to redeem myself in Tim's and Eddie's eyes and bust up that black cloud blocking the sun in Wilmington.

"How far along is she?" I asked Lee Walker as he opened the door.

"Twenty-eight weeks," he replied.

At least that was what I thought he said. He might've said twenty weeks. Or thirty-eight. I didn't know—I was so amped up and already had tunnel vision on finding my patient and bringing new life into the world. "You're a white cloud," Julie had said to me during my rotation in the labor and delivery ward. I desperately wanted it to be true now.

Through the living room and down the hallway, Lee led us past the nursery and master bedroom. I carried the first-in bag in my hand and such hope in my heart. I couldn't wait to hear the newborn's first vigorous cry, announcing itself to the world.

But when I found Mia Walker, she was kneeling in a puddle of blood on the bathroom floor with her baby, who was dead.

There are some moments working as a paramedic that you can never prepare yourself for. No classroom scenario can ready you for the shock and horror of seeing a lifeless, premature baby, with its fused eyelids, small size, and tiny fingernails. In all honesty, I froze. But Tim recognized this immediately and jumped in before the Walkers had any sense of delay. "Hello, ma'am," he said gently, placing a hand on her shoulder. "My name is Tim and I'm a paramedic with the Los Angeles Fire Department and we're here to help you. I am so sorry for your loss . . ."

"I'll get towels," Eddie said, heading out to the ambulance. He returned with blankets and towels, and cut the umbilical cord. Tim and I helped Mia to her feet and assisted her to the gurney. Lee kissed his wife's forehead and took her hand.

But what to do with the baby?

I was horrified at the thought of using a red biohazard bag. But what else was there?

"Hold this," Eddie said, handing me a small pink plastic basin. It was shallow and kidney shaped. Eddie lined the bottom of the basin with a clean white towel, then gently placed the baby inside and covered it with another towel. I handed the basin back to him and Tim and I wiped up the bathroom floor. The last thing the Walkers needed would be to return home from the hospital to find bloodstains on the linoleum.

Mrs. Walker didn't watch any of this. Her eyes were closed. She was right next to us on the gurney and, yet, miles away. Her skin was pale and she looked as if her whole body was raw nerve. As I applied the blood pressure cuff to take a preliminary set of vital signs, I worried even the small squeeze on her arm would cause her the greatest pain.

"You're going to feel a little pressure on your upper arm," I said softly, hitting the "autoinflate" button on the cardiac monitor.

Mia didn't respond.

"Kaiser Hospital in Harbor City is our closest hospital," I said to Mr. Walker. "We'll meet you there."

Lee kissed his wife again and we wheeled her into the hallway and past the master bedroom. Past the nursery with the crib and new changing table with a wreath above that said, "Welcome Home, Baby!"

Mia's eyes stayed closed and, for a few steps, I shut mine, too.

People lose their past when a parent dies. But when a child dies, they lose their future. I knew I could do little to alter the difficult days ahead for Mia Walker—but I could affect the ten minutes she was in our ambulance. Therefore, I reclined the gurney to the exact angle she found comfortable, dimmed the lights in the patient compartment, turned up the heat when she started to shiver, and told Eddie, who was driving, "Let's go slow and easy on the bumps!"

"Copy that," he replied. "ETA six minutes."

Eddie was already driving with the greatest care, but I said it aloud so Mia knew that LAFD was doing everything we could for her.

The lights in the ER were bright and, as we wheeled Mia in that morning, tears began to stream out of her still-closed eyes. She'd dreamed of arriving at the hospital under such different circumstances.

"You guys can go to bed four," the nurse said as we passed registration.

We lowered our gurney to the height of the hospital bed and Mia eased herself over. Her eyes were still closed and we held her hands to help her. I brought her an extra pillow. Tim and Eddie brought heated blankets. Lee Walker arrived and we grabbed him a chair. We apologized to the Walkers again for their loss. And just before we left, Mia opened her eyes and took my hand. "Thank you," she whispered. "You guys were so nice."

August

Trial and Initiation

Prior to my arrival at Station 38, Los Angeles mayor Antonio Villaraigosa and the city council had cut LAFD's annual budget by $88 million. Station 38 had lost a ladder truck and the firefighters who'd staffed it. The residents of Wilmington, fearing the city was closing the fire station, took to the streets, waving signs and shouting, "Save lives! Save Station 38!"

In Wilmington, you could see the positive effect Station 38 had on the community by the way the children stopped by on their way home from school, and how the firefighters were invited to attend charity relays, benefit dinners, and award ceremonies. And you could see it when Scott Lewon, an athletic guy in his midfifties, stopped by the station with his wife, Anna, to thank Tim and Eddie for saving his life.

Tim and Eddie had responded to the Lewons' home late one night a few months prior because Scott was feeling anxious and short of breath.

"It's probably just stress from work," Scott had told them. "I don't need to go to the hospital."

Tim and Eddie performed a full assessment on him—vital signs, a 12-lead ECG, blood sugar, pupil check, and physical exam—the whole bit. And everything was within normal limits. But he was still anxious and sweating and struggling to breathe and there was nothing emotionally going on that might've explained it, either.

"You need to go to the hospital right now," Eddie told him. "I'm worried you may have a pulmonary embolism."

A pulmonary embolism (PE) occurs when a blood clot forms a sudden blockage in the lungs. A number of conditions can cause a PE, but they are often the result of a long period of immobilization such as a long flight or recovering after surgery.

"I'm fine," Scott replied. "I'll follow up with my doctor in the morning."

Since Scott was alert and oriented, Tim and Eddie couldn't force him to hop in the ambulance—they could be held liable for kidnapping if they did—so they kept insisting he go. But Scott remained steadfast in his refusal, speaking in short, winded sentences. Finally, Tim had slammed his clipboard down on the table and yelled, "God damn it! If two paramedics say you should go to the hospital, then you should go!"

Scott reluctantly agreed and they quickly loaded him up.

"What did the doctors find?" Tim asked, as we all stood on the sidewalk outside the station.

"I had a pulmonary embolism, all right," Scott said. "And it had divided into two arteries. The doctor said I would've been dead in fifteen minutes."

"No kidding," said Tim, shaking his head.

"A saddle PE," added Eddie. "That's almost always lethal."

Scott shook Eddie's and Tim's hands to thank them. "Your bedside manner wasn't the best," he joked, "but you saved my life."

Following my eleventh shift, I felt I was reaching a critical point in my internship. Though the comments at the bottom of my daily evaluation had once said things like, *No extension requested,* and *No red flags at this point,* the notes now said things like, *Lacking experience,* and *Calls need preceptor intervention to take shape.* Had my performance dropped? Or had Tim's and Eddie's expectations risen? I knew they'd soon decide whether to extend me past twenty shifts—or fail me—and a good barometer of progress would be when (or if) they started letting me give radio reports to the hospital. That would mean I was competent in my patient assessment and treatment and ready for the added responsibility of notifying the hospital about the patient we were bringing them.

Eddie continued his ceaseless criticism. "When you're doing something, you're not talking," he lamented one day. "And when you're talking, you're not doing anything. You have to multitask!" Along with this, he was constantly yelling at me to "get it done." In fact, he said "get it done" so much, I was beginning to think it was more a philosophy than a phrase to him. I got that, but I still felt like Eddie's constant griping was getting in the way of me finding my flow on the calls. And yet, I also recognized that the very same traits that made him a harsh preceptor were what made him an amazing paramedic. He was an expert at picking out problems—but it certainly didn't make internship any easier.

As Tim had suggested, I was beginning to believe that Eddie had it out for me. For instance, I was certain I'd set that oxygen bottle atop the gurney after we'd moved the patient to the ER bed, and convinced that he'd placed it back on the floor to test me. I found it a little unfair if he'd really set me up like that, but I also couldn't overlook the teaching point—as the lead paramedic, I had to take ownership of every aspect of every call. I decided to give up hoping for praise from Eddie. After all, back on shift two, he'd instructed me to only "verbalize what is broken and needs fixing." So now, rather than hoping for praise, I had a new goal with Eddie—keeping him quiet.

It wasn't only Eddie riding me, though. Tim had also begun hammering me about my patient interactions. "I want you to take acting lessons on your next four-day break and learn compassion," he said on shift eight. Since I'd always prided myself on my bedside manner— and been complimented on it—his criticism felt especially biting. *I* knew my compassion was there, but it got hidden under the mechanical assessment style that stress and nerves brought out in me.

Tim's and Eddie's comments made me wonder—were my attempts to perform the "perfect" assessment getting in the way of doing the *correct* assessment? In my case, I thought the answer was likely yes. When I was on scene, I was often thinking about all the "right" questions to ask so I could show Tim and Eddie the extent of my knowledge. Yet when I asked one question, I was already thinking about the next one, so I wasn't truly listening to the answer. I wasn't present with my patient and, instead of having a good flow, the call became mechanical and forced. I would miss vital information or end up asking the same question multiple times.

Case in point: I'd been assessing a woman with abdominal pain during one call and, to show my preceptors what a great medic I was, I asked her all the pertinent questions relating to abdominal pain, including the date of her last menstrual period. Which would've made a lot of sense, if she hadn't been seventy-four years old. "Really? Her last menstrual period?" Eddie hollered behind the ambulance after the call. "If you'd asked if there was a chance she could be pregnant, I was going to fail you on the spot!"

Despite my struggles, I was learning a lot about the job—and myself. I'd always been one to lead by example, but as a paramedic I discovered that that leadership style wasn't effective on scene—I needed to vocalize specific details about the patient's condition to the crew. I also realized that the perfectionist in me didn't like to delegate tasks, lest I appear lazy, but delegating tasks like taking vital signs or holding a patient's head in spinal immobilization were crucial so that I could stand back and run the call, keeping the momentum moving forward.

During some moments on scene, however, when I felt I was finally connecting to the flow of the call, it was the greatest feeling. And I knew being a first responder was right where I wanted to be, helping to restore the flow—of oxygen in the lungs, fluid in vessels, life to the body.

The last and perhaps the most important thing I realized was that I had to fight to keep control of the call and prevent Tim and Eddie from stepping in. I needed to prove to them, and to myself, that I could run the call. But maybe the reason I was struggling to live up to their expectations, it occurred to me, was because I hadn't observed Tim or Eddie run a call.

On my twelfth shift, we decided I'd watch Eddie run a call, but it had to be the right call. It couldn't be the thirty-three-year-old man who was dehydrated, surrounded by empty liquor bottles, who said, "There's no one to blame for any of this. I drank myself into oblivion." Nor could it be the eighteen-month-old baby with a tiny laceration on his head, or the fifty-year-old man with mild abdominal pain. It had to be a critical call. But when would it arrive?

"No idea," said Tim. "Sometimes we sleep through the night at Station 38."

Despite this, I sensed that call would arrive as surely as the sun would set over Catalina Island and teenagers would blaze up the Cali Kush, a potent strain of weed, in MacArthur Park; as surely as lines would form behind felt ropes outside Hollywood nightclubs and prostitutes would strut the concrete catwalk of Long Beach Boulevard. And it came, all right. Around ten p.m., we were dispatched for an unconscious fifty-six-year-old male with ineffective breathing. As we hurried to the rig, Eddie said, "This one's mine."

We found the man hunched over, chin to chest, in the back bathroom of a halfway house.

"Hey, wake up," Eddie said, tapping him.

The man didn't respond and Eddie quickly checked his pupils with a penlight. "Constricted. This guy's high as a kite," he announced. "Let's get him out of the bathroom."

Nick, Carlos, and Bryan quickly moved in, patting down the man's pockets for any heroin needles before carrying him to the gurney.

"Let's put him on oxygen," Eddie said, as the firefighters buckled the man in, "and I'm going to start an IV now, check blood sugar, and give Narcan."

Narcan was the drug used to reverse a narcotic overdose. As I watched Eddie nail the IV on his first attempt and push the medication, I couldn't help but think that watching him run a call was art in motion. He was, at once, fully attentive to his patient but also directing his team. He was completely present in the moment and, yet, also planning three steps ahead. Was Eddie a bit highstrung on scene? Without a doubt. But I realized he was working fast not so much because of where his patient was now—breathing with slow, shallow respirations—but where he was headed: respiratory failure. By working five to ten minutes ahead of his patient and treating the worst-case scenario, Eddie was assuring that his patient never arrived there.

"Always push Narcan slow," Eddie advised as he gave the medication. "You want to raise their respiratory rate but also keep them somewhat sedated."

"How come?" I asked.

Eddie told me that if you bring a heroin addict out of their overdose too quickly, they'll likely get combative. "They just paid good money for their high and now you've taken it away."

"But you saved their life," I protested.

Eddie shook his head in such a way that let me know I had no idea the lengths people would go to get their high.

I couldn't help but think how Eddie's skills were a combination of several different careers: he possessed the critical thinking skills of an ER doctor, the compassion of a nurse, the leadership skills of a great coach, and a police officer's expertise in scene management, and he handled his equipment like a competent mechanic. There was a choreography and grace to the call that even reminded me of a conductor.

"How did you know it was an overdose?" I asked as we arrived back at the station.

Eddie said that sometimes the location where a patient is found can point you to his or her condition. "If you're called to someone who's unconscious in a bathroom or car, always consider an overdose."

"Got it," I said, jotting it down in my notebook.

"Any questions?" Eddie said, starting off.

"No, sir," I said, calling after him. "Thanks for the demonstration!"

Later, as Eddie walked into the television room, the doors closed behind him like the swinging double doors of a Wild West saloon, and I had no more doubts—that was how you got it done.

Inspired by Eddie's example, I tried to emulate him for the rest of the shift, making strong decisions, verbalizing my treatment plan, and replicating his overall leadership style.

"I'm not sure if he's altered because he's been drinking or because he got kicked in the head," I said about a fifty-year-old man who'd been assaulted, "so let's backboard him, get going to the hospital, and I'll start an IV en route." And as we loaded the man, his face bloated and bloodied, onto the gurney, an LAPD officer said, "Did you know a boot can be considered assault with a deadly weapon?"

On the next call, around 2:15 a.m., we responded to a sixty-six-year-old female found unresponsive in her bed.

"Let's get some lights on," I said, marching into the bedroom, "and move these cats out of here!"

There must've been fifty cats in the house and the stench of the kitty litter made my eyes tear up even through my safety glasses.

The woman had a history of high blood pressure and diabetes, so I quickly delegated tasks to Carlos and Nick. "Let's get her on oxygen and the cardiac monitor and take a blood sugar."

"Blood sugar is low," Bryan said moments later.

"Okay, we'll start an IV and push dextrose," I announced.

"Don't say it—do it," said Eddie. "Faster."

I had Nick hold the woman's arm straight while I started an IV. I missed my first attempt. Nailed the second. And then I pushed dextrose and the woman woke up, became alert and oriented, and didn't want to go to the hospital. I advised her of the risks and consequences of refusing transport and she still didn't want to go. I repeated her vital signs and checked her blood sugar again. It was within normal limits by then. Tim made the woman a sandwich and said, "You should eat this because that dextrose will wear off fast."

"Are you sure we can't take you to the hospital?" I asked again.

"I am sure," the woman replied.

We had her sign a release of liability form. She scribbled her name and thanked us for our help, then said, "Aren't my cats darling?"

"They sure are," I replied—eyes tearing, nose running—as I navigated through the furry living room maze. "Don't hesitate to call us back out if anything changes and you start to feel worse."

Back at the station, Tim congratulated me. "That was a good run for you," he said, climbing the stairs toward the bunkroom. "Keep it up."

As always, Eddie had nothing good to say about the run. But, as he went up to bed, I realized he also hadn't had anything bad to say, either.

Progress.

On Saturday, August 24, I sat down with Tim and Eddie for my fourteenth shift major evaluation. Once again, Tim started with my strong points—I had a solid work ethic; I arrived for each shift prepared and well rested; my attitude was good; and I acted professionally at all times. "Since you performed well on the cardiac arrest, we've also given you '3s' for ECG interpretation, intubation, end-tidal CO_2 monitoring, and CPR," he said.

When Tim paused and looked down at his written comments, I knew bad news was coming. "We were hoping to have you giving radio reports to the hospital by now," he confessed. "But we don't feel you're ready. You're still struggling with patient communication, leading your team, and scene management."

As much as I wanted to, I couldn't argue. On one call, I'd released the engine back to the station because I assumed I wouldn't need their assistance, only to discover the patient was severely dizzy and dehydrated and couldn't walk. Tim, Eddie, and I easily handled the situation but I couldn't make the same error in the future when I was working alone in the back of the ambulance. Also, at times I was still robotic on scene and used medical terminology that the patients didn't understand. For example, we'd been dispatched to a run-down apartment building for a pregnant woman having contractions so, naturally, I'd asked about the onset, frequency, and duration, and if her "amniotic sac had ruptured and if she'd had any 'bloody show.' "

"That woman had no idea what you were talking about!" Tim fumed. "Keep it simple and just ask if there's any water or blood running down her leg!"

"Based upon calls like these, we don't feel comfortable starting you on the radio," Eddie said.

When I heard this, I realized there was virtually no way I'd be out in twenty shifts. But what did I expect? Internship was never easy, and anyone who said otherwise wouldn't pass a polygraph test. In fact, in addition to Crook, I'd heard that three more students from Class 36 had now failed out due to poor field performance.

As Tim and Eddie finished up, I presented a strong front, but deep down I was disappointed. I promised them I'd work hard to improve in all the areas they'd mentioned and start being a leader and communicating more.

"You might start praying more," said Eddie.

Following my fourteenth shift evaluation, it was an unusually quiet afternoon and evening at Station 38. Was the black cloud above Wilmington finally dissipating? I was hopeful, but at 4:39 the following morning, Dean Molino, who lived on West Anaheim Street, went to wake his six-year-old daughter, Jolita, and found her in the middle of an uncontrolled seizure.

The call woke me from a deep REM sleep, jolting my heart from resting to racing. As we sped to the scene, I suspected it was a febrile seizure, triggered by a high fever. They were quite common in children below the age of six, were rarely life-threatening, ended quickly, and often only happened once. But as I opened the door, Mr. Molino literally threw Jolita into my arms. She was still in her purple-footed pajamas, decorated with blue and yellow flowers, but her eyes were rolled back into her head and her arms and legs were rigid.

"She's still seizing," I announced, racing to the couch and setting her down.

Since febrile seizures rarely lasted longer than a minute or two, this was a true medical emergency, so we jumped into our pit crew approach to get the job done and save her life. Nick put Jolita on high-flow oxygen and I directed Tim to start an IV.

"Got it," he said, pulling out a catheter.

"What do you need from me?" asked Eddie.

I told him to get Versed, a sedative used to stop seizures, from the lockbox in the ambulance. "Done," he said, hurrying out.

I quickly checked Jolita's ABCs—her teeth were clenched and drool dribbled out the corner of her mouth. Her back was arched, her skin pale, and she couldn't take a deep breath.

I grabbed the Broselow tape—a color-coded tape that measures a child's height and provides the accompanying weight and medication dosages—from the first-in bag and laid it out beside her. She fell into the "blue" box, typical for five-to-six-year-olds who weighed between nineteen and twenty-two kilograms. I called out the appropriate dose of Versed. "Slow IV push," I said, "and we can go internasal if we can't get a line."

The Broselow tape also listed the type of equipment that should be used to intubate and the level of shock dosage for defibrillation if a pediatric patient went into cardiac arrest. Sadly, as Jolita continued to seize, such a scenario seemed imminent. "Seizure deaths are hypoxic deaths," Mr. Wheeler had told us in one of his lectures. "And kids go into cardiac arrest secondary to respiratory arrest." Jolita had likely been seizing before her father found her, seizing as he called 911, and seizing as we responded from Station 38 to the scene. You didn't need med math to know that was a long time.

"How's my O_2?" I asked.

"Her pulse oxygen is rising," Nick said.

"I've got an IV," said Tim, inserting his needle into a red sharps container.

Eddie returned with the Versed and handed me the syringe. I cleansed the administration port of the IV and slowly pushed the medication, keeping an eye on Jolita. Would her rigid, doll-like arms become human again?

Jolita continued to seize for twenty seconds and then her extremities relaxed and her eyes rolled back into the sockets, to hide behind heavy lids.

"What now?" Eddie asked.

"Rapid transport to closest pediatric medical facility," I replied, picking her up.

I told her father we'd meet him and his wife at the hospital. A parent could ride in the ambulance on a less-critical call, but, with this one, we needed space in case Jolita went into cardiac arrest.

"Good," Eddie said. "Get it done."

En route to Harbor-UCLA, I continued Jolita on oxygen and reassessed her vital signs. Her skin had "pinked up," her blood pressure and pulse were good, and I didn't see any oral trauma or incontinence from her seizure. But we weren't out of the woods yet. Jolita was still sleepy and lethargic. Was this the normal postseizure, postictal (sleepy) phase? Or had she sustained permanent brain damage?

"Come on, Jolita," I said, gently tapping her shoulder. "Wake up for us."

My words had no effect. Her eyes weren't tracking me and her body swayed with the motion of the ambulance.

"Two minutes out!" Eddie yelled from the driver's seat as we exited off the 110 Freeway near Harbor-UCLA.

I quickly switched the oxygen tubing from the house tank in the ambulance to an oxygen bottle on the gurney and took another set of vitals. Jolita was still out of it.

"Should the postictal phase last this long?" I asked Tim as we parked at the hospital. "I hope she doesn't have brain damage."

Tim told me the postictal phase could last up to thirty minutes in some patients.

"Come on, Jolita," I said again as we unloaded the gurney. "Wake up for us."

Despite the early hour, the parking lot at Harbor-UCLA was teeming with ambulances and police cars. It was always rush hour there.

As we wheeled Jolita toward the ambulance entrance, I noticed her arms and legs begin to move slowly, as if she were crawling back into her skin for the first time.

"Hey, Tim," I said excitedly, "I think she's coming around."

Doctors passed us wearing white lab coats with stethoscopes dangling over their shoulders. As they did, Jolita's eyes subtly began following them and squinting in the bright light.

"I think she's coming around, too!" Tim exclaimed.

What we saw was a six-year-old girl in her purple-footed pajamas, becoming more alert and oriented. But what Jolita saw was a bunch of firefighters pushing her on a tall gurney. Suddenly she burst into tears and my heart danced. I'd never been so happy to hear a child sob in my life! Crying meant not only that Jolita had an airway and was breathing, but also that she was awake enough to realize she was at the hospital, in the company of strangers, and her parents weren't present. I was so thrilled I damn near started crying myself!

Already I couldn't wait to get off shift and text people to say that today we'd saved the life of a six-year-old. But not only that— we'd also saved all the potential that resided within Jolita. I was overjoyed, but now Jolita was really bawling and people were beginning to give us strange looks, so Tim unfastened her seat belts on the gurney and took her into his arms, and there it was—a firefighter in yellow turnouts cradling the child he'd just rescued. I know of no better image of America's commitment to its people.

When we arrived at the pediatric ER, a team of doctors and nurses waited. The nurses wore lavender scrubs and had panda and monkey face snap-ons for their stethoscopes. Tim set Jolita down on a bed. I gave a report and the nurses rushed in to do their assessment. Jolita continued to improve, her vital signs remained normal, and she was laughing by the time we left. There was a good chance she'd make a full recovery.

Later, as I cleaned up the back of the ambulance, I didn't feel so bad about the prospect of being extended to twenty-five shifts. Sure, it meant five more days with the potential to fail out, but it also brought more opportunities to help people, saves lives, and learn from two seasoned paramedics. Bringing Jolita out of her seizure was a strong field save but, as the final month of paramedic school arrived, I didn't pretend to think the sky above Wilmington was suddenly filled with blue sky and white clouds. For the moment, I was just happy it wasn't raining.

September

Becoming a Street-Smart Paramedic

That September was the bloodiest month of the year in Wilmington. It seemed to begin around midnight on the night of September 10, when Socorro Fimbres, twenty-five, allegedly got into a fight on the 1100 block of R Street. Punches were thrown and Socorro was shot in the chest. He was raced to a local hospital by his friends, but bled out in the parking lot and was pronounced dead at 12:23 a.m.

The *L.A. Times* Homicide Report—an interactive map, database, and blog—listed the basic details of Socorro Fimbres's death, under which grieving family members and friends wrote condolences in the reader comments section . . . and then became engaged in a war in the comments with strangers who took offense at the Homicide Report becoming a memorial to "gangbangers," and so on.

I wondered what was behind the uptick in violence that September. We responded to several traumas and assaults, as had the other shifts at 38 (including one where a fifty-five-year-old man was shot to death by police after attacking them with a sword). Certainly, the battle for the guns, drugs, and money played a role, but what was the source of the rage? Was it the claustrophobia of refineries and industrial junkyards pressing in from all sides? Or maybe it was just that rotten smell always hanging in the air, the stench so bad on some nights that kids started crying and couldn't fall asleep. Maybe it was all those things . . . or maybe it was about one word.

Respect.

In Los Angeles, California, respect has a value greater than currency. Here, people may steal for money, but they kill for respect. But how do you gain respect? And once earned, how do you hold on to it? What do you do, for instance, if you're playing pickup basketball in Venice Beach and that guy who dunks on you holds on to the rim for an extra second, pointing and mocking? Do you take his legs out from under him next time he leaves his feet? How do you react when that rival gang member dares to exit off the 110 Freeway in your neighborhood? Do you roll up alongside him on the Slauson Avenue exit—the one that winds around in a two-lane circle so you can get off a good shot without any witnesses—roll down the window, and yell, "You better recognize!" And what about that paramedic you called for abdominal pain who says you only have the flu and don't need to go to the hospital? How do you respond when your friends, sitting next to you on the couch, start laughing?

I heard a story once about a paramedic who responded to that exact call in one of L.A.'s worst neighborhoods. While the housing projects in cities like New York and Chicago rise up as towering apartment buildings, in L.A. they spread out in two-story apartments that encompass city blocks. To reach one of the 1,054 units in the Nickerson Gardens complex in Watts (or a complex like Imperial Courts or Imperial Downs), you often have to take a right, then a left, then another right, then a left, then a right, and soon you have no idea how you got in—how you'll ever get out—and your handheld radio is suddenly coming in all static.

So there the paramedic was, telling the boy with abdominal pain that he didn't need to go to the hospital. The paramedic informed the boy in front of his friends that he likely had gastritis and explained that this was the condition responsible for the nausea and vomiting most people labeled "the flu." However, the only diagnosis the boy heard was "wimp-itis," and there his friends were, smirking. The boy made the paramedics take him to the hospital anyway.

The following day, paramedics were called to the same apartment complex. To the same floor, for a patient the same age and with the same chief complaint. But the unit number was different. This time, they were called to the apartment at the end of the hallway, where the light was broken and it stayed dark even in the daytime. Since the call had come in as "mild, nontraumatic abdominal pain," dispatch had sent only the ambulance, staffed by two paramedics. And since it was the following day and there'd been a shift change, that also meant two new paramedics, who had absolutely no idea what they were walking into.

They knocked three times.

"He's in the back room," said the man who answered the door. He had fat red laces running through his Converse All-Stars. Baggy red shorts. He wore a red shirt and a red rag clung to his head.

The paramedics walked in and heard the door shut behind them . . . and lock. Unbeknownst to them, it was the boy from the day before. When they turned, they saw him, surrounded by five members of the Bloods street gang.

"Is this him?" one hulking guy asked, gesturing to the lead paramedic.

The boy looked the paramedic over. He wore the same black boots and blue station uniform. He had the same badge from the same department . . . but the nameplate was different. And the face.

"Nah," the boy said. "Ain't him."

The front door opened. "Get the fuck outta here," the man said to the paramedics.

Tim and Eddie were always adamant about treating our patients with decency and dignity. "We must respect people who don't respect themselves," Tim said to me as we sat in the kitchen on my seventeenth shift.

Just then, I heard the double doors of the kitchen swing open and Eddie entered. His heels dragged slightly as he walked, like spurs, as he took a seat at the table next to Tim. We'd arranged to meet that day to make a final determination about extending me to twenty-five shifts. I'd had two shifts since my shift fourteen evaluation and we'd run calls for dizziness, a fall, acute anxiety, a pregnant woman with abdominal pain, and a fifty-five-year-old man, not breathing and pulseless, whom I determined to be beyond resuscitation due to rigor mortis under Policy 814.

"Your knowledge base is good," Eddie conceded, "but you lack consistency and are still having trouble on scene extracting information from patients."

"You're always professional with patients," Tim added, "but we feel you're not producing answers leading to a treatment plan fast enough."

I didn't disagree. On some calls, I felt as if my assessment was getting in the way of my patient rapport. On other calls, my interaction with the patients was good, but my assessment was slow.

"Imagine the calls as visits instead of chief complaints," Tim said, reminding me of the advice Captain Turner had given me before. "That will help you stay connected with your patients. When you get on scene, immediately check their radial pulse. That will connect you with them instantly. Think of the patient's wrist as the steering wheel and their eyes the road."

"And then engage them and work fast to get the information you want," added Eddie. "Unless you realize nothing will ever be handed to you as a paramedic, you'll spend the next six years fumbling around."

"We think with time and more experience that you'll be able to complete the program," Tim said. "But right now, we feel you'd benefit by being extended to twenty-five shifts."

I'd expected this, as I hadn't been on the radio, but I was still disappointed to hear the news. Now my back was up against the wall. Earlier that week Ms. Davis, our program director, had sent out an e-mail with details about graduation. *September 30th, 2:30 p.m. Family and friends welcome. Dessert and reception to follow ceremony.* If I was cleared in twenty-five shifts, I would finish my field internship in the morning and could attend graduation with the rest of Class 36 that afternoon. If Tim and Eddie extended me to thirty shifts, I could still attend graduation, but I wouldn't receive a diploma, which, to me, would ruin most of the fun in attending. I felt there was no other option—I *had* to finish internship in twenty-five shifts.

I told Tim and Eddie I'd do my best to improve.

It was about that time that a fifty-seven-year-old man at an industrial park in Harbor City began feeling a crushing weight in his chest.

As the tones sounded, I promised my preceptors that I'd focus on scene management, connecting with patients, and my communication. I was such a conscientious student. But Tim and Eddie shook their heads and looked at me like I was missing something crucial. What was it?

"Until you walk in the door knowing you're the man that's going to save that patient's life," Eddie said, "you will never be a paramedic."

It was attitude.

"Let's go," Tim said, starting for the rig. "It's time for you to join the ranks!"

We were responding as a medical aid in Harbor City, and we found one of the firefighters from Station 85 waiting for us by the first-floor elevator.

"The patient's on the third floor," he told me as the elevator ascended and numbers beeped. "They got you doing radio reports yet?"

"Not yet," I replied, tightening my grip on the cardiac monitor.

"When he's a *paramedic*, we'll put him on the radio," Tim added. Fair enough.

As the elevator doors opened, I noticed three firefighters huddled around a middle-aged man seated at his desk chair. He looked anxious and pale. I also noticed the paramedic from 85 appeared to be the same guy I'd blazed past without taking his report on the shooting call on my first shift. Now was my chance to not only help a man with chest pain but also rectify that error.

As the paramedic saw me approach, his eyes tightened defensively and he gave me a look that said, *Not this guy again* . . .

But I had my pen and a small pad of paper ready to take a report—my apology.

"Hello, sir," I said, walking up, "what's going on today?"

The paramedic turned his gaze down to the monitor.

"Can I please get a report?" I asked.

He looked back up at me. "This is Doug," he began, somewhat reluctantly. "He's a fifty-six-year-old man . . . Chief complaint chest pain . . . Unprovoked that came on suddenly when he was seated at his desk . . . We've given him 162mg of aspirin . . ."

As he continued, I scribbled everything down. "Thank you for the report," I said when he finished.

Just then, one of the firefighters handed me a 12-lead, as another relayed Doug's vital signs. The 12-lead showed no ST elevation and his vitals were stable.

I quickly introduced myself to Doug and said, "We'll be taking over care and transporting you to the hospital." Then I turned to Tim. "Let's give him a round of nitro and get him loaded up." This would ease the workload on Doug's heart, open up his vessels, and reduce his chest pain.

Moments later, as we arrived at the ambulance, the firefighters from Engine 85 helped me load the man into the back and the paramedic from 85 asked if there was anything else I needed.

"I'm good," I replied. "Thanks so much for your help."

"Not a problem," he said, nodding. "We'll see you on the next one!"

En route, I started an IV, rechecked Doug's vital signs, administered another two doses of nitro, repeated my initial assessment of his ABCs, and eased his anxiety by talking to him. By the time we arrived at the hospital, Doug was feeling much better and all signs pointed to angina, a predictable pattern of chest pain, versus an acute heart attack.

After we dropped Doug off in the ER and left the hospital, Tim applauded my efforts. "You took a good report from the medic on scene, assumed care immediately, and got the patient going to the hospital quickly and followed the chest pain protocol perfectly."

Instead of feedback or advice, Eddie had a question: "We have the oxygen bottle back there?"

I looked around—it wasn't on the gurney.

Eddie slammed on the brakes. "Are you kidding me?"

I told him that the oxygen bottle was back in the airway bag. "I saw it on the hospital floor after giving my report, so I grabbed it!"

Eddie let out a triumphant cheer. Hit the gas and then cranked up the radio—Creedence Clearwater Revival's "Born on the Bayou."

"Well, all right!" he howled, smiling. "There's hope for you yet, son!"

I tried to keep that sense of momentum on my next shift. I approached a man hunched over the steering wheel of an old white Toyota Camry on Island Avenue in Ghost Town. Was he alive? Had he been shot? Stabbed? Or had he been sucking down a carbon monoxide cocktail courtesy of the tailpipe for the last hour?

I set my equipment down and knocked on the window. Nothing. So I opened the car door and leaned him back in his seat. He took one gasping breath and then didn't inhale again for eight seconds.

"Airway's clear," I announced to Tim, "but his respiratory rate is very slow. Let's get him out of the car!"

As we moved the man, I realized we'd run a call on him before, on my fourth shift. His name was Gonzalo and he'd called us out that morning to his methadone clinic, complaining of shortness of breath. Methadone is a synthetic drug that acts on the same receptor sites as heroin and morphine to reduce pain and produce a feeling of euphoria. The medication is prescribed to people with a history of narcotic abuse to lower their dependence on illegal drugs and all the ensuing side effects, such as crime, sharing needles, and prostitution. When I asked Gonzalo that morning when his shortness of breath started, he told me hours before he went to the clinic.

"How come you didn't call us out then?" I said.

"Because I needed my methadone," he replied, proving that, for some, "H" comes before anything else in the ABC flowchart.

As we moved Gonzalo to our gurney that afternoon, I discovered his pupils were pinpoint, along with his altered level of consciousness and slow breathing rate. *Bathrooms and cars,* Eddie had said.

We quickly put him on oxygen, to reverse the respiratory acidosis of a narcotic overdose, and loaded him into the back of the ambulance to start an IV. Gonzalo's upper extremities didn't look too different from the mannequin IV arms we'd used at paramedic school—they were tough and scarred with track marks from a thousand needle sticks. Nonetheless, I tied off my tourniquet, found a vein, and nailed the IV.

As I did, Gonzalo's brother and sister-in-law pulled up in a Chevrolet Blazer. Turned out, Gonzalo had overdosed in front of his house.

"He's using again, isn't he?" his brother asked, rushing up.

"We don't really diagnose patients in the field," I replied. "But I'm confident we can bring him out of this."

"Oh, thank God," his brother replied.

What none of us knew at the time, however, was this would be Gonzalo's last night on earth. None of us knew that Gonzalo would spend the night in the hospital and then, after being discharged early the following morning, he'd wander into traffic on the Pacific Coast Highway and get hit head-on by a semitruck. I wouldn't be on shift, but other paramedics from Station 38 would respond and find him in traumatic full arrest. "Everything was crushed like seashells," the medic would tell me. But before Gonzalo left the hospital to die, our job was to make sure he arrived at the hospital alive.

When Tim handed me my daily evaluations from shifts seventeen through nineteen, I was relieved to see positive feedback. *Much better assessments . . . Getting rhythm and starting to act like a paramedic . . . Improving with experience and getting involved with patients on a personal level . . . Questions coming earlier and findings are more concise . . . We are going to start him on the radio if this keeps up!*

I was thrilled, but before I left the station Tim reminded me my next shift would fall on September 11.

"Something will happen," he said, ominously. "Somewhere."

September 11, 2011, was the tenth anniversary of the worst attacks on U.S. soil. For me, the day began as it had every September 11 since 2001: I awoke feeling sad and slightly nauseated as I recalled the horrific images from that tragic day. Every anniversary of it was an occasion for prayers and remembrances, but, when we gathered outside Station 38 for a moment of silence on the morning of my twentieth shift, it was also an occasion for a dedication. As I stood facing the flag—its red, white, and blue triumphantly lighting up a gloomy, gray morning—I dedicated my twentieth shift to the 343 fire personnel and the thousands of other first responders, members of the military, and civilians who lost their lives that day. Perhaps the city of Los Angeles wouldn't ask that I serve my country in the heroic manner on that day in which those first responders had served theirs. But if it did, I hoped that I could summon the same kind of courage to rush into the smoke and help those in need.

Following the moment of silence, we spent some time driving around the streets of Wilmington and the Harbor, patrolling the area for any unusual activity. It was the first time we'd done such a patrol, but, rather than feeling uneasy, I felt such pride to be interning with LAFD. Since the Los Angeles and Long Beach ports were a major potential terrorist target—shutting them down would cost the U.S. economy an estimated $1 billion a day—we had our eye out for any strange behavior, but we also wanted to show a presence in the community. On that day of national tragedy, we wanted to remind the people of Los Angeles that we were there to protect them. And, should there be any terrorists in the Harbor, we wanted to prove to them once again that they could bomb our boats, tear down our towers, and put a plane into the Pentagon, but they'd never break the spirit of the American people.

Around noon, we stopped for lunch at a little Mexican restaurant on Avalon Boulevard, famous for having burritos the size of small sleeping bags. But our waitress had just set down our plates when the tones sounded: *Engine and rescue . . . a sick person.*

As we pulled up to a weekly motel with an empty pool and a flashing "Vacancy" sign, we found Evelyn Palmer hurrying toward the ambulance. She was a heavyset woman wearing a gray sweatsuit and walking a green oxygen tank behind her like a small puppy. Clear tubing ran from the tank, under her arm, and up her torso, before thinning into two prongs, one for each nostril. As I took in the scene, a number of things immediately crossed my mind. She was ambulatory—that was always a good sign—but the oxygen bottle suggested a history of chronic obstructive pulmonary disease (COPD), asthma, or another respiratory condition. Being overweight, it was likely she also suffered from high blood pressure or diabetes. And while she didn't appear to be in any major distress, the fact that she was walking out to meet us with some urgency suggested something was wrong.

"Hello, ma'am," I said, climbing out of the ambulance. "How can we help you today?"

"I'm just not feeling right," Evelyn said, looking concerned.

"Do you have any pain?" I asked.

"No."

"Feel short of breath?"

"Not more than usual."

The day was hot and sunny and I noticed Evelyn's brow beginning to moisten so I told Tim I wanted to load her up and continue my assessment in the back of the parked ambulance.

"I'm invisible," Tim replied and I realized I'd reached that stage of internship where my preceptors stayed quiet on scene. In many ways, the silence was more daunting than the yelling.

"That sound good, Evelyn?" I asked. "Get you out of this hot sun and into some air-conditioning?"

"Oh, I'm probably just being dramatic," she replied as I assisted her onto the gurney.

I checked Evelyn's ABCs, vital signs, and blood sugar in the back of the ambulance and found nothing unusual, but I had a bad feeling in my gut. Evelyn was still anxious and I couldn't find a cause.

"Any recent surgery, long flights, or extended periods of sitting?" I asked, trying to rule out a pulmonary embolism that may have originated from a deep vein thrombosis (blood clot) in her leg that traveled to her lungs.

"Nope," she said.

"Have you been sick recently? Any nausea or vomiting?"

Evelyn shook her head.

"Anything stressful or emotional going on?"

"No, sir."

As I asked Evelyn about her medical problems, I caught a scent of something.

"I have insomnia, diabetes, high blood pressure, and COPD," she said, wiping her brow with a tissue.

What was it? I recalled from our cardiology block that women over the age of fifty—and especially those with diabetes—can present with very mild or atypical symptoms for a heart attack. I was also concerned that Evelyn appeared to be sweating more than ever, despite being in the air-conditioned ambulance, and none of my calming measures were working.

"You will learn to smell death," Dr. Larmon, director of the Center for Prehospital Care, had said.

I decided to take a 12-lead ECG. "Just to cover all my bases," I said, applying the electrodes, "I'd like to take a detailed look at your heart."

I looked over at Tim. He sat in the captain's seat with a blank expression on his face, but looking and listening to every word.

Once the electrodes were on, I asked Evelyn to hold still and I hit the "acquire" button. The cardiac monitor took a few moments to analyze the rhythm before printing the six-second strip. I quickly scanned the morphology of the ECG tracing and then the monitor interpretation further confirmed my suspicion:

Acute MI Suspected

I handed the strip to Tim and yelled up to Eddie: "We've got ST elevation on the monitor. Let's get going—Code 3!"

Eddie pulled out into traffic, blasting the air horn before busting a U-turn toward the PCH and gunning it toward the 110 Freeway.

"Am I going to be okay?" Evelyn asked as I quickly gave her aspirin to chew.

And how to answer this question? Tell her the absolute truth—*you're having a heart attack!*—and risk raising her anxiety level and, by extension, increasing her body's oxygen demand and the workload on the heart? I decided not to lie to Evelyn, but I also wouldn't go into great detail. "To be honest, ma'am, your heart is showing some distress on the ECG monitor," I began. "But we're doing everything we can and the hospital is going to take great care of you."

Evelyn sat back in her seat. "Oh, no . . ."

I put a hand on her shoulder to calm her. "You just try to relax, ma'am, and think of a happy place," I said. "I'm right here by your side and I'm not leaving."

As Eddie blasted the horn again at a semitruck that wouldn't pull over, Tim piped up, suddenly visible. "You need any help?"

I heard him, but was too focused on Evelyn to answer. "You sure you're not having any chest pain?" I asked again. "If so, I can give you nitro."

"No pain," she said again.

"ETA five minutes out!" Eddie yelled from the front.

"I'm here if you need me," Tim added.

"No worries," I replied, "I can get it done . . ."

And as I spoke these words that had so often been said (and shouted) at me, I suddenly understood their sacred meaning. There was an obstacle on every 911 call, and "getting it done" meant rising to the challenge; not shying away from the moment, but plunging into the fire. "Getting it done" meant embracing the obstacles—whether they appear on scene or within yourself—and using them as a stepladder to make your ascent. "Getting it done" meant you let go of excuses and, instead, did everything in your power to save someone's life. *The best way out is through*—I finally understood.

Amen!

Just then, Tim handed me the radio. "Here you go, kid."

"Go ahead with your run," the nurse at Harbor-UCLA said.

I froze, shocked to see something so long wished for suddenly in my hand.

"Go ahead with your run," she said again, more insistently.

I brought the radio to my mouth, my hand shaking with nerves, and tried to replicate one of Tim's reports: "Good afternoon, Harbor base," I began. "This is, um, Rescue 38 Paramedic Grange—"

Tim corrected me from the captain's chair. "Paramedic *Intern*."

"Paramedic Intern Grange," I added. "We have, um, a fifty-one-year-old female whose chief complaint was anxiety . . ."

"Go ahead, Rescue 38," the nurse sighed, already frustrated.

What followed was, perhaps, the worst radio report in history, which, of course, was broadcast throughout the entire ER: "We were, um, called to a weekly motel for a fifty-one-year-old female complaining of anxiety . . . Um, we found her in mild distress and, ah, she had ST elevation on the monitor so, um, we gave her aspirin and, ah, she chewed that right up . . . Um, we didn't give her nitro because she denied any chest pain, ah, but I certainly can if you'd like . . ."

On and on it went, with very little rhyme or reason but a lot of pauses, "ums," and "ahs." The nurse had to remind me to give her vital signs, as well as the patient's medical history, allergy information, and what medications she was on.

"Copy that, Rescue 38," she said a moment later. "I'll tell the STEMI team to expect you. You can obtain IV access and give nitro if the patient develops chest pain and recontact us if the patient's condition changes. Harbor base out."

The moment I hung up, I handed the radio to Tim and immediately returned to Evelyn. "How do you feel right now?" I asked. "Still no pain?"

Evelyn shook her head no. "Hanging in there . . ."

Evelyn's condition hadn't improved by the time we arrived at the ER, but it also hadn't worsened. As opposed to shift one, when I'd been shocked to find a team of doctors and nurses waiting, this time I was ready, and, unlike on the radio, my voice was strong and confident when I gave the report. After transferring Evelyn to a bed, I placed a hand on her shoulder and said I hoped she felt better. She thanked me and smiled. Since we'd caught her heart attack early, the doctors informed me she'd likely survive.

When I turned, I found Tim standing with the nurse, chuckling. "I counted about thirty 'ums' during your report," he said.

"I was giving the nurse a chance to write everything down," I joked.

We all had a good laugh at that.

Tim told me not to worry. "We'll teach you more about radio reports on your next shift," he said, "but the bottom line is you're on the radio now and acting like a paramedic."

I found Eddie waiting out behind my ambulance. But instead of scolding me, he shook my hand. "Nice job on catching that STEMI," he said. "That easily could've been missed."

We wouldn't run any more calls that shift and the tenth anniversary of September 11 would come and go in Wilmington without incident. Not only had catching that "silent MI" in Evelyn put me on the radio, but it was also the first run where I received "3s" in every category on my daily evaluation. But just as things were beginning to come together for me, Wilmington was about to fall apart. Socorro Fimbres had been shot the night before. More bodies were about to drop . . . and Station 38 would be dispatched to pick up the pieces.

September

Radio Reports

I was finishing up my ambulance inventory late in the morning on my twenty-first shift when Tim and Eddie came out to teach me about radio reports.

"The purpose of a radio report is to paint a picture for the nurse or doctor," Tim began. "You're trying to sell them on your chief complaint and treatment."

"As you saw during your clinical shifts, the ER staff is busy," added Eddie, before pausing to hawk tobacco juice into an EMS exam glove. "You need to get their attention with your report. If your patient is critical, you need to make sure that gets communicated."

Tim and Eddie told me the end result of a good radio report is always improved patient care. If the patient is critical, the nurse will be more apt to grant you orders for any medications or procedures you've requested and, when you arrive, they will have an open bed and team of doctors ready.

"First step is to give your rig number and what type of call it is," Tim said. "Tell them if it's medical or trauma."

"And then wait for them to respond and clear you to start talking," Eddie added.

From there, I'd follow with the scene location—*private residence, business, roadway*—and then give the patient's age, sex, and chief complaint. After that, I'd go into how the patient presented—*supine, standing, seated, lying unresponsive*—and in what degree of distress—*mild, moderate, severe*—I'd discovered him or her.

"Then go into a brief history of present illness or injury," Eddie explained, "followed by the patient's medical history, allergies, and medications."

Next, I would relay the patient's vital signs—pulse, blood pressure, respirations, skin signs, level of consciousness, lung sounds, appearance of pupils, blood sugar, and ECG rhythm—along with informing the nurse of any interventions we performed and the outcome. Did the patient improve? Deteriorate? Or was there no change?

"The last piece of the radio report consists of informing the nurse what the ETA to the closest hospital is," said Tim, "and then whether you'd like to transport there or reroute to a different facility."

"If you'd like to get an order for a medication or procedure, the end of the report is also the place to ask for it," said Eddie.

When I finished taking notes, I realized that my last five shifts would be the hardest of internship. I would now be in charge of all aspects of the call, including radio reports. All throughout paramedic school, I told myself things would get easier—as a way of coping with the pressure—but I realized it was a mathematical equation that only built in responsibility and complexity. I told myself, too, that being a licensed paramedic would be easier than interning with two preceptors constantly harping on you, but Tim quickly squashed that idea. "You think it's scary now? Wait until you're alone in the back of the ambulance and your patient is crashing."

As calls started coming in, I struggled to stay one step ahead of Tim and Eddie for the remainder of that week—using talking as a "treatment" to calm a thirty-year-old woman having a panic attack; asking for a breathing treatment of albuterol the moment I heard another patient wheezing; and making the difficult decision not to treat a woman whose "one" chief complaint was something like: chest pain, shortness of breath, a fainting episode, full-body pain rated ten of ten in severity, and feeling "like I'm dying."

"You're not going to treat her?" Eddie asked as the firefighters loaded her into the ambulance.

I told him there wasn't anything I could treat. "Her oxygen level is normal. Her blood pressure is good, so she doesn't need fluid," I said. "Her chest pain is more pleuritic in nature than cardiac. Her ECG and blood sugar are normal. I don't see any sign of trauma and she doesn't appear to be in any pain. If she was, I'd see it somewhere— in skin signs, increased heart rate, or her face grimacing."

Early in my internship, I would've likely uptriaged and gone lights and sirens to the hospital, but in this case my provider impression was that she was stable despite her answering yes to all my questions. (She also had a history of schizophrenia, which might've explained her answers.)

Eddie agreed, but pointed out that I should avoid asking leading questions. "Instead of asking if she has chest pain," he said, "say something like, 'Do you have pain anywhere?' and let her tell you."

The calls that night went well and I felt in the flow, but, while I'd fortified the walls of the dam over the past few shifts, I knew the reservoir of doubt was still there. Thus, as we responded to a private residence for a forty-year-old man complaining of chest pressure, I tried to work fast and confidently. I did a quick assessment, took vital signs on scene, and then gave aspirin and nitro and initiated rapid transport, calling in my radio report en route.

"This is Rescue 38, Paramedic Intern Grange with a medical run," I began, reading off a note card I'd prepped for myself.

"Go ahead, Rescue 38," the nurse said.

"We were called to a private residence for a forty-year-old man, weighing approximately 260 pounds, complaining of chest pain. We arrived to find the patient in moderate—"

Tim motioned for me to slow down.

I stopped and took a breath. "We arrived to find the patient seated in his living room chair, alert and oriented, in moderate distress. The patient described the pain as a 'dull ache' and said it was unprovoked and began twenty minutes ago. Initially he rated his pain a six out of ten in severity and he states nothing makes the pressure feel better or worse."

As I spoke, I noticed Tim nodding slightly—a good sign.

"Patient denies any shortness of breath, nausea, or vomiting, and my physical assessment revealed no neck vein distention, trauma, or swelling of the feet or ankles," I continued.

Tim put up a hand for me to pause—miming the nurse scribbling down notes—and then, like a choreographer, pointed for me to continue.

"Patient has no remarkable medical history," I said, starting to have fun. "He denies any allergies and only takes daily vitamins. His vital signs are all within normal limits; he has clear lung sounds; his skin signs are pink, warm, and dry; and his 12-lead ECG showed no ST elevation."

I took another breath.

"At this time we are following the chest pain protocol and the patient states the oxygen and nitro have helped and now rates his pain around a four out of ten. Our ETA to your facility is . . ."

"Three minutes!" yelled Eddie, listening up front.

"Three minutes," I said, noticing I'd arrived at the end of my note card. "How do you copy?"

The moment of truth had arrived. Had I effectively conveyed the patient's condition? Would the nurse agree with my assessment findings and treatment plan?

"C-o-p-y t-h-a-t, Rescue 38," the nurse replied in that elongated way people do when they're both talking and writing frantically. "No questions or orders. We'll see you in three minutes. Harbor base out."

Tim nodded and gave me a thumbs-up. Four shifts left.

What's the craziest thing you've ever seen?

It's the one question EMTs and paramedics are asked all the time and, over the course of internship, I often found myself pondering it as I drove home through morning rush-hour traffic. Sure, the shootings, overdoses, and accidents were intense but they were never the craziest. To me, the most insane calls were always the ones when people, in the throes of sickness or death, were filled with regret about the way they'd lived their lives. *I wish I hadn't drank so much . . . I wish I'd had the courage to follow my dreams . . . Traveled more . . . Stayed in touch with my friends . . . Hadn't worked so hard . . . Didn't let that good girl go . . . Spent more time with my kids while they were growing up.* At times, the ambulance resembled a four-wheeled confession booth and, driving home from Station 38 each morning, I was always reminded of the fragility and beauty of life.

So that September 17, I decided to forgo the usual studying I did on my days off and celebrate my birthday—technically on the eighteenth—with my family. We spent the afternoon at the pool in my apartment complex, swimming, eating cake, and opening presents. A celebration was also going on back in Wilmington. Three blocks of Avalon Boulevard had been closed off and transformed into a street carnival, with inflatable slides, spinning teacups, a Ferris wheel, and food stands. The scent of cotton candy and the sound of children's laughter rose up in the air, but, around noon, shots rang out nearby and Miguel Munoz fell down, dead.

The shooting occurred two blocks from the carnival, on the 700 block of East L Street. According to the *L.A. Times* Homicide

Report, Munoz was walking when an unknown person walked up and shot him multiple times. Was this shooting retaliation for the September 10 killing of Socorro Fimbres? The double stabbing I'd responded to the night before? It was impossible to tell, but, as my alarm woke me at five o'clock the following morning for my twenty-second shift, it seemed that bodies were falling like dominoes in Wilmington and no one knew when they'd stop.

Around the same time I clicked off my alarm, Rescue 38 was responding to a call on the 1100 block of West Anaheim Street for a boy with severe stab wounds. Minutes earlier, Rogelio Alvarado had been standing with friends when a guy asked for a drink. Alvarado declined and the man stabbed him. Alvarado stumbled to a nearby courtyard, where he collapsed. He was rushed to the hospital, but later died.

As the day started, the ominous black cloud feeling returned and I wondered when the violence would end. In Los Angeles, it's not uncommon for one gang to retaliate for a killing with another killing—an eye for an eye—which then causes the first gang to retaliate for the retaliation, and on and on it goes.

Thankfully, my first two calls that shift weren't gang related. One was a ninety-seven-year-old woman with wheezes complaining of shortness of breath, and the other—if you can believe it—was a thirty-seven-year-old man who'd called 911 over a nosebleed. But when we dispatched to Cruces Street for an unknown medical, we were about to confront the harmful effects of gang violence head-on.

As I unloaded the gurney outside a two-story apartment advertising one month of free rent, I didn't like what I saw in my scene size-up. People in the yard and on the balcony, some crying, some arguing, and others pleading and questioning. All the stages of grief were present—denial, anger, bargaining, depression—except acceptance. Whatever these people were mourning, it was still too raw for that last one.

"What are you thinking?" Eddie asked as we pushed the gurney into the crowd, surrounded by the firefighters from the engine.

"I'm not liking this scene," I whispered.

"Me neither."

Just then, a woman in her early twenties hurried over. Her cheeks were tear streaked and dark circles hung under her eyes. "I'm so glad you're here," she said. "I'm Tina."

"What's going on?" I asked. "Does someone need an ambulance?"

Tina explained that she'd called because her little brother had been killed the previous night by gang violence in another part of L.A. and her father didn't know yet. She explained her father would arrive at any moment and she was worried he'd have a heart attack when he heard the news. "I wanted you here to make sure he is okay," she said. "Please help us!"

Suddenly everyone in the yard fell silent. Her dad had arrived. He was a short, skinny man with his flannel work shirt tucked into faded jeans and an extra loop punched into his belt to make it fit. You could tell by his face he had no idea why everyone—including himself—had gathered there. As his eyes found us, Tina waved him over.

"What do you want to do?" Eddie asked me. "Stay or go?"

That was easy—there was no emergency. No chief complaint and nothing to treat. This call was exactly like one Eddie had once told me about, when a guy had called 911 because his cable TV wasn't working. Then again, Captain Turner, Tim, and Eddie had always preached the importance of talking to people.

"I want to stay on scene and help Tina out," I said.

"But there's no complaint," Eddie said, testing my resolve.

"True," I said, "but that doesn't mean LAFD can't provide a service."

Eddie nodded. "Good answer!" he said. "But let's do it inside the ambulance."

I informed Tina of our plan. She nodded and took her dad's

hand, leading him to the ambulance where his world was about to be destroyed.

Tina's father—Armando—sat on the gurney and her brother, Joaquin, took the captain's chair. Tina and I sat on the bench seat. Eddie listened from the front seat and Tim stood at the back ambulance doors. Armando didn't know English so Tina spoke to him in Spanish.

"*Papá, te llamamos porque tenemos unas noticias muy graves,*" she began.

"*Qué?*" he replied, looking at me. "*Por qué están aquí los socorristas de emergencia?*"

"*No vas a creer lo que ha pasado, Papá,*" Tina said, choking back tears. "*Es tan horroroso.*"

I couldn't understand a word, but I knew exactly what they were saying. It was clear in the tone of their voices and body language.

"*Qué pasó?*" Armando asked.

Tina broke down. "*José murió anoche.*"

"*Qué?*"

"*Sí, fue herido con arma blanca,*" she said. "*Está muerto!*"

"*Está muerto!*" Joaquin said suddenly from the captain's chair, holding his head in his hands.

Armando stared into space for a few moments. I could see the information slowly travel down from his head into the rest of his body, distending the veins on the sides of his neck and stiffening his shoulders. And when it reached his heart, he physically recoiled and let out a terrible wail. It was almost too painful to watch.

A moment later, Tina nudged me. It was time. I pulled out the BP cuff and pulse oximeter from the side pocket of the monitor.

"*Estaba preocupada, así que llamé a los socorristas de emergencia para examinarte,*" she explained to her father. "*Te importa si te hace unas pruebas?*"

Armando nodded and I wrapped the BP cuff around his trembling arm. I hit "autoinflate" and then slipped a pulse oximeter over his fingertip and checked his other vitals—pulse, respiratory rate, and lung sounds.

"All of his vital signs are normal," I told Tina a minute later.

"*Qué?*" Armando asked.

"Everything looks good," I said loudly, as if raising my voice would help him understand. "Your heart is stable."

Of course, we all knew that wasn't true.

"*Te sientes capaz de entrar ahora, Papá?*" Tina asked.

Armando nodded and glanced at the ambulance door.

"*Porque si necesitas ir al hospital—estos señores te pueden llevar,*" added Tina.

"*Al hospital, no,*" Armando said with a whimper.

Tina turned to me. "He can go inside now."

I removed the BP cuff and oxygen probe. "Anything else we can do for you today?"

Tina shook her head sadly and thanked us for helping her family.

"Not a problem," I said, as we assisted them out of the ambulance.

The rest of the family waited in the front yard. Eddie radioed dispatch and cleared us from the call. As we drove away, I saw Tina and Joaquin walking with their father. They were on each side of him, holding him up.

"When a part of the heart dies, another part takes over to keep it beating." Dr. Atilla Uner had said during our cadaver lab in January.

Automaticity.

With one exception, I received all "3s" on my twenty-first shift, and I tried to maintain my performance in the shifts that followed, blending my scene management, patient assessment and treatment, leadership skills, and communication into one cohesive flowing call.

A thirty-three-year-old woman hyperventilating: "You feel as if you need more oxygen but what your body really needs is carbon dioxide," I said, coaching her, "so I want you to breathe slowly in through your nose and out through your mouth . . ."

A forty-three-year-old woman who'd had a hot flash: I printed out the 12-lead rhythm strip, scanning it for any signs of ST elevation or distress. "I put you on the cardiac monitor just to cover all my bases," I told the woman, "but I'm happy to say everything looks normal."

A forty-five-year-old male found under a tree, intoxicated, with a low blood pressure: I started an IV, connected the tubing to a bag of normal saline—which would rehydrate him—and opened it up wide.

On a later shift, as I helped Tim prep dinner by chopping vegetables, he informed me that I was doing a great job and would pass internship. "You made the team."

"Yes!" I said, high-fiving a carrot on the cutting board with my chopping knife.

But there was a caveat. "Unless we get called out to a seven-year-old with her face blown off and you say, 'I can't treat her,' you will pass," Tim added. "That would be like one of the guys on the engine rolling up to a structure fire and saying, 'Sorry, fellas, I'm not going in.' Our *job* is to go in."

"The best way out is through," I said, happily.

"Exactly."

Just then, the front doorbell rang and I rushed out to answer it. Eddie joined me, sliding down the fire pole from the bunkroom upstairs.

It was a young woman with her two children. One was a fourteen-year-old girl and the other, an eight-year-old boy. Through broken English, she said she'd come to find out if her oldest son was alive. There'd been more violence in the Harbor and now family members were out searching for loved ones. Her son had been stabbed the night before and the last thing she'd seen was him being loaded into an LAFD ambulance. *Not again*, I thought. I couldn't bear to tell another parent their child was deceased.

Eddie explained he'd worked that night and Rescue 38 hadn't transported him. "But let me call Station 85 and see if they know anything."

Eddie ducked into Captain Turner's office and called the Harbor City station, leaving me alone with the family. The daughter stood biting her nails nervously. It was clear she knew what was going on. Her little brother had no idea—he was staring at the engine and wondering why the firefighters' turnouts were scrunched up atop their boots like that.

"When a call comes in, the firefighters jump into their boots and pull up the turnouts," I said, mock demonstrating. "It's faster that way."

The door to Captain Turner's office opened and Eddie returned. His blank expression gave me no indication which way this would go.

"I spoke to a paramedic at Station 85 in Harbor City and they transported a patient matching the age and description of your son," he began.

The woman's eyes widened and she straightened with hope. "Is he okay?"

Eddie smiled. "I'm happy to say he's alive."

"Alive?" she exclaimed.

"He's alive and recovering well," Eddie replied. "He's at Long Beach Memorial hospital."

The woman called over her son and then she and her daughter shook our hands, thanking us profusely.

We ran only one call that night—a twenty-four-year-old male

with a parole cuff around his ankle, complaining of shortness of breath. I gave him an albuterol breathing treatment for his wheezes. We took him to the hospital.

In the morning, Tim reminded me I was to cook dinner for the crew on my twenty-fifth shift. "If we don't like your meal, we'll extend you," he said.

I believed him.

That night, I boarded a red-eye flight to Boston. I'd been planning to attend my cousin's wedding in New Hampshire for months and had assumed I'd be finished with internship by then. But since I'd started in the field late and been extended to twenty-five shifts, I was left with a tough decision—skip the wedding and break a commitment I'd made to family, or skip a shift and risk threatening Tim's and Eddie's opinion of my commitment level. I brought the question to them with some trepidation.

"Go to New Hampshire!" Tim said without a second thought. "We'll finish your last two shifts when you're back."

"Family always comes first," Eddie added.

As the plane left the tarmac that night, the L.A. basin spread out under me in an endless colorful grid. My eyes instinctively found the coast and followed it down to the towering cranes of the harbor, where I swore I saw the flashing lights of Rescue 38. While the relationship of ambulances arriving and departing from the hospital reminded me of LAX, Tim—being a waterman—naturally thought of fishing. He often referred to getting a 911 call as "catching a run."

"Some days are busier than others," he told me one night as we washed the ambulance. "But we never come home without a catch. We always make somebody's day a little bit better. And that's why I'm always smiling when I scrub the decks."

As my plane rose higher and veered east, I lost sight of the harbor and closed my eyes. Did I really see Rescue 38 that night? It was doubtful. I was sleep deprived, exhausted, and likely on the verge of hallucination. But one thing was certain—I'd been away from Station 38 for less than twelve hours and I already missed it.

It's been said that you can't go home again, but that doesn't mean you can't drive by the fire station that inspired you as a boy. The Newfields Fire Station in New Hampshire looks today exactly the same as it did all those years ago. Only the pickup trucks and names on the turnouts have changed. I had a wonderful time back in New Hampshire—the cozy antique towns, scenic beaches, and tasty lobster rolls—but a large part of me stayed focused on paramedic school. When I found myself seated at the wedding reception next to my cousin Jamie Morse, an ER physician, I asked for his thoughts on paramedics. Jamie attended medical school at McGill University, completed his residency at Yale, and is now the assistant chief of emergency medicine at Anna Jaques Hospital in Newburyport, Massachusetts.

"The first person on the scene is often the paramedic," he said, pointing out how the critical hour (or as I knew it, the golden hour) was when "quick, directed care can make the most important difference in the health and sometime even life of a critical patient." Paramedics, Jamie noted, "initiate the direction of the patient's care and rapidly provide the stabilizing treatment needed in the critical moments before hospital arrival."

"How do paramedics drive your care as an ER doctor?" I asked him.

"I rely on a good patient evaluation and report to rapidly integrate my team with the patient's clinical scenario, provided treatment, and current condition," he explained. "This allows us to build off of the work done in the field and hit the ground running in transitioning the patient from the prehospital care into the critical hour of emergency department care. Without that boost, we would be receiving a much sicker patient with no immediate insight into the clinical details of their case."

Jamie also added that sometimes a paramedic brought in the only available history on a patient (or important objects, such as medication bottles from home) and provided key information that would be otherwise unobtainable.

"It is that kind of access to information, identification of critical conditions, and initiation of lifesaving stabilization of the most critical of patients that makes paramedics a pillar in the emergency care I provide," he said.

"Cheers to that," I said, raising a glass.

We toasted, then hit the bar for another round. Three days later, I found myself at a grocery on the corner of Sepulveda and Imperial Highway, shopping for my final meal at the station.

I prepared to cook my final meal with the same diligence and methodical planning that I'd extended to my proficiency drills.

My twenty-fourth shift had gone well. I'd returned from New Hampshire and jumped right back into a seizure call, a fainting episode, and a forty-year-old male who told us he'd called 911 so he could go to the ER where he'd get a free bus token that he could use to visit his mom in Long Beach.

"I'm not lying. His chief complaint was initially a lack of transportation," I told the nurse on my radio report. "But during my assessment, I found his blood sugar was elevated, so I've started an IV to give him some fluid and dilute the excess sugars in his system and reverse his dehydration. At this time, he is resting comfortably on our gurney . . ."

Tim and Eddie awarded me "3s" on all the calls and, at the

bottom of my daily evaluation wrote: *Working well on calls and running all aspects of the incident.*

When I got off shift at six thirty a.m. following my twenty-fourth shift, I drove straight to the grocery store to prep for my final meal, Chicken Marbella, one of the most popular dishes to come out of the renowned *Silver Palate Cookbook*—and, equally important, a meal I could prepare mostly in advance, on my day off. The last thing I wanted to be doing on my final shift was running cardiac arrest calls and worrying about cooking at the same time.

Control what you can control—it even applied to cooking.

After I finished shopping, I picked up the suit I'd wear at graduation the following day, then spent the afternoon quartering chicken, peeling garlic, cutting olives, and chopping parsley. I mixed these last three in a large bowl with oregano, red wine vinegar, olive oil, prunes, capers, and bay leaves, added the chicken pieces, and coated them in sauce before putting them in the refrigerator to marinate overnight. The dish was virtually finished, so the only thing I'd have to do on shift was arrange the chicken in a shallow baking pan, add a brown sugar and white wine glaze, and bake it. I'd complement the Chicken Marbella with rice pilaf, a salad, and Cookie Dough ice cream—Dreyer's, not Breyers.

When I was done prepping my meal, I found myself at my desk with *Emergency Care in the Streets.* I'd instinctively gone to my desk because, after all, that had been my routine every evening for the last nine months. But I shut the book a moment later. It was five p.m., the waves were head high, and there were still two hours of sunlight left. I grabbed my surfboard and drove to the beach.

September

Graduation

The last shift of my internship ended with us staging outside a known gang house in Harbor City. There was a twenty-eight-year-old man inside named Isaiah, who, according to his neighbors, might have a history of schizophrenia. They also said he might have a gun and want to shoot everyone. They'd seen him running around the yard earlier that day with a knife and called 911. When the police arrived, they found the doors locked, shades drawn, and no one answering when they knocked and yelled, "Police! Open up!" Engine 85 from Harbor City was also on scene and we'd been called out as a medical aid. We rolled up to find a bunch of police officers, firefighters, and Isaiah's girlfriend walking up the driveway toward the house. She'd decided that now—with the house totally surrounded by law enforcement officers—was the perfect time to profess her undying devotion to her boyfriend.

"I love you, baby!" she yelled, walking closer.

"Move away from the house!" a police officer yelled.

"I'll never leave you, baby!"

"Move away from the house now!"

The woman paused long enough for a cop to race out and grab her.

The first part of my twenty-fifth shift had been unusually slow. Earlier that day, we responded to a day care for a two-year-old who'd fallen and bumped his head. He hadn't lost consciousness, and I didn't see any significant trauma during my physical assessment, but we transported him nonetheless as a precaution. After that call, we treated a forty-year-old woman complaining of mild abdominal pain. Even though neither call required a paramedic intervention, I was still attentive and methodical in orchestrating every aspect of each run. After all, my struggles during field internship were rarely about performing a specific skill like starting an IV or intubation, they were about scene management, communicating with my patient, and directing my team.

When the tones sounded again early that afternoon, Tim told me to stay behind and start cooking my final meal.

"You sure?" I asked, as the engine rolled out.

"You bet," Tim replied, hopping on the ambulance. "You earned it!"

I watched them depart down the street, glad to be on my last shift, but also yearning to hop aboard and run more calls. I wandered back into the kitchen and preheated the oven to 350 degrees, arranged the chicken in a single layer in a shallow baking pan, spooned on the marinade, and set it in the oven to cook. The chicken took an hour to cook. All the guys were back from the run by then, so I quickly set the table, removed the rice from the stove, tossed the salad one last time, and reached for the station intercom:

"Dinner. Ten minutes," I announced.

My dinner was a huge hit. The firefighters all heaped second servings onto their plates and, of course, there were the inevitable jokes:

"His cooking is like his assessment," Eddie said. "He just throws everything at it."

"Quick, I need an emesis bag," added Bryan.

In between the jokes, the guys glanced up at *Wedding Crashers*, once again playing on the flat-screen television in the kitchen. When I caught myself watching, I instinctively dropped my head.

"You can watch," said Tim, chuckling. "You're at that point now."

Following dinner, I hopped on dishes and then wandered out onto the apparatus floor to wash Rescue 38 once last time. As I moved my towel over the letters "LAFD"—written in white over red paint—I knew I'd miss the rig almost as much as the crew. There is an affection between EMTs and paramedics with their ambulance, no different from a pilot's love of his plane or a sailor's soft spot for his ship. After all, Rescue 38 had not only brought us safe passage to calls, but had also transported us back to the station and, by extension, back home to family and friends. After I finished washing Rescue 38 that evening, I gave it a good gleam of wax.

That was when we got called out to Harbor City.

As we hopped off the ambulance, we took cover behind the engine with the firefighters from Station 85. The night was hot and sticky and you could taste the rotten smell from Wilmington's refineries. We waited ten minutes—all amped up—but there was no movement inside the house. We waited silently for another ten minutes. Still nothing. Ten minutes after that, we were standing behind the engine, casually chatting about the Angels and Dodgers. Were we ready to respond? Of course. But there was no point in staying in a constant state of stress; when it came time to engage we would simply hit the "get it done" switch inside ourselves and do just that.

"The front door is opening," a police officer suddenly yelled.

There was the clicking sound of a dozen police officers taking aim.

A moment later, Isaiah stumbled onto the porch with his arms held high in surrender. He was a disheveled man in his late twenties with wild hair, a dirty white T-shirt, and holes in his jeans. It was clear he'd lost the ability to care for himself.

"On your knees now!" a police officer yelled.

Isaiah dropped to his knees as the police officers advanced from both sides before tackling him to the ground and quickly securing his hands behind his back. Moments later, they waved us over.

Isaiah would be put on a seventy-two-hour "5150" involuntary psychiatric hold—and perhaps go to jail—but first he'd need to be cleared medically in the emergency room and that was where we came in. Up the driveway we pushed the gurney and, when we arrived at his side, I quickly assessed him. He had no deficits to his ABCs and was alert and oriented. A few abrasions, with strawberry-like designs, dotted Isaiah's elbows from his scuffle with police, but other than that he was fine. We loaded him up and got going to the hospital. En route, I learned he played guitar and we talked music. Led Zeppelin, Jimi Hendrix, and Jack White.

Was I friends with Isaiah? Hell no. Was I angry that he'd potentially risked the lives of his neighbors and the police officers and firefighters who responded that night? Without a doubt. But I didn't show any of this. "The paramedic badge means we don't judge," Mr. Wheeler had said.

I talked about the guitar with Isaiah that night because it eased his fear and paranoia, kept his vitals stable, and prevented him from becoming combative—rock-and-roll was good patient care.

We cleared from the hospital around nine thirty p.m. and it was about that time that shots rang out on Blinn Avenue in Ghost Town. *So my last shift is going to go down like this?* I thought as we raced to the scene. My pulse skyrocketed. But as we arrived on scene, an LAPD officer immediately cleared us.

"No patient found," he yelled. "You're good."

Tim shut off the emergency lights. I removed my exam gloves and safety glasses and my pulse dropped to normal. We cleared back to the station. Ate ice cream and then gathered in the TV room to watch another movie.

About that time the tones went off again, and we were dispatched to a shooting in Harbor City with multiple victims. On went my exam gloves and safety glasses. Sweat dotted my brow and my heart raced once again.

We pulled up to an apartment building bathed in the red, white, and blue lights of police cars and fire trucks. A captain from Station 85 hurried over to meet our ambulance.

"There's only one patient and we got him," he said, as his paramedics rushed a young teenager out on a gurney. "You guys can clear."

Tim again deactivated our emergency lights and we headed back toward Wilmington. My pulse returned to normal and I took off my gloves and safety glasses once more. Back at the station, we watched ESPN for a bit and I was in bed by midnight. The cool air and roar of the AC unit put me to sleep right away but, at 3:47 a.m., I heard *bang-bang-bang* right outside the station. I lurched up, expecting the station lights to blaze on and phone to start ringing. Was it gunshots? A nine-millimeter Glock pistol? Or a car muffler? Minutes passed. No lights. No phone. I lay back down and fell back asleep.

I woke up at 5:45 a.m. and quickly packed up my bedding and cleaned out my locker. When the oncoming crew arrived, I took my equipment off the ambulance and placed my boots, turnout pants, helmet, and ballistic vest back into the station locker. Tim, Eddie, Captain Turner, Nick, Carlos, and Bryan all met me on the apparatus floor to say good-bye. As I shook their hands and thanked them profusely, they gave me their final words of wisdom regarding working as a paramedic and a firefighter, if I pursued that as well.

On getting hired by the fire department: "Always be improving yourself," said Bryan. "Test everywhere and never give up."

On the nature of the job: "We're in a bad situation all the time," added Nick. "That's just what we do. But remember, it's not your emergency."

On treating patients: "This job is about talking to people," said Captain Turner. "Think of the calls as visits and always make a connection."

On visiting Station 38 in the future: "Come by anytime," said Carlos. "You know where to find us."

Tim and Eddie walked me to the door. "Thank you both so much," I said. "I couldn't have asked for better preceptors."

Eddie congratulated me and advised me to always keep learning as a paramedic. "Always find a better and faster way of getting it done."

"Amen to that," I replied.

Tim shook my hand and said to visit the station if I ever wanted to learn more about the firefighting aspect of the job. "Come ride out on the engine—throw some ladders and we'll introduce you to the equipment."

I thanked Tim and Eddie again. Hopped into my car and slowly pulled out. I rolled down the window and waved. And just before I was out of earshot, Tim yelled out one last order:

"Give me a call and we'll surf!"

As I left the station that morning, something in me wasn't ready to go straight home, so I drove past my apartment and parked on the corner of La Cienega and Lennox Boulevard, just outside LAX. During the nine months of paramedic school, whenever I'd needed to de-stress, I'd gone to that spot to watch the airplanes and catch my breath. And perhaps it was the perfect place, for paramedics inhabit the landing strip of life and death—one passenger arriving, while another departs—and such was the heartbreaking beauty of the world.

As I leaned against my car that morning, airplanes stretched across the sky like a string of white Christmas lights and I felt such pride to live in America. Even as I stood there, I knew there were firefighters and EMTs, paramedics and police officers, spread out all across our great nation, getting it done, and I made a wish that each and every one of them got home safely.

As the sun rose, bathing the runway in gold, I thought back to the first day of classes at UCLA. Hard to believe that nine months earlier, we'd all walked into the Walter. S. Graf Center as EMTs— full of passion and promise, but also some doubt and uncertainty— and now here we were in September, pushing meds, intubating patients, starting IVs, and saving lives as paramedics.

In less than seven hours, Class 36 would assemble for the last time at graduation. There would be commencement speeches by Dr. Baxter Larmon and Program Director Heather Davis, and Brian Wheeler would have the entire auditorium in stitches with his humor. We would laugh about botched skills stations with Justin McCullough and field internship foibles with Nanci Medina. Lewis's paramedic rap song would draw resounding applause, and a hard-working and humble student from Manhattan Beach named Robinson would be crowned valedictorian. Diplomas and hugs would be handed out, and last but not least, we'd unveil our Class 36 plaque. But before any of that, there would be a few hours of something hard-won and found in short supply over the last nine months.

Sleep.

UCLA–Daniel Freeman
Paramedic Education Program

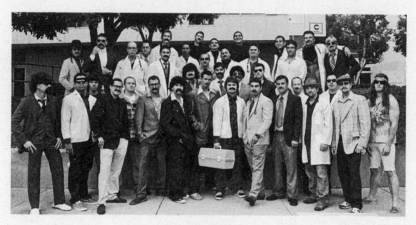

Class 36
September 2011

Afterword

On a sunny June afternoon in 2014, Edward Herzog, sixty-one, stood with his wife, Annie, on the Old Faithful boardwalk in Yellowstone National Park watching the famous geyser erupt. They'd been married for over forty years and had always dreamed of visiting Yellowstone, and that day, the world's first national park seemed to be rewarding them for their efforts: a herd of bison lumbering across the road had greeted them as they entered the park; hot springs, mud pots, and thermal vents had bubbled and steamed—as if to say hello—as the Herzogs toured the Fountain Paint Pot Nature Trail; and now, Old Faithful geyser was shooting water and steam 150 feet into the blue sky. When the majestic show was over, Edward and Annie followed the boardwalk to the Old Faithful Lodge for lunch and a coffee. But as they walked out of the cafeteria afterward, Edward suddenly grew short of breath. His eyes rolled back in his head and he fell to the ground.

I was working as a paramedic with the National Park Service

when I heard the call go out over the radio: *"Paging Old Faithful EMS, please respond to the Old Faithful Lodge for a sixty-one-year-old man in cardiac arrest."*

I was doing ambulance inventory at the time, but I threw my clipboard aside, raced to the front cab of the ambulance, and hit the ignition. Clicking the garage door open, I activated the emergency lights and pulled out.

The Old Faithful Lodge sat a short distance away from the ranger station, but it might as well have been five miles. The parking lot was jammed with tour buses, RVs, minivans, pickup trucks hauling trailers, and dozens of people hurrying toward the Old Faithful visitor center. I navigated through the lot with the ambulance lights flashing and my siren and the air horn blasting.

As I drove, I heard additional park rangers responding over the radio. At Yellowstone, I often drove to 911 calls alone in the ambulance and was then met on scene by law enforcement rangers who shared collateral duties as EMTs and paramedics. They assisted with patient care, documentation, driving the ambulance, and, on black cloud days, delivering bad news. That afternoon, the whole cavalry was coming, which was a good thing, because as I parked beside the Old Faithful Lodge, it was absolute pandemonium. The lodge was swarming with tourists lining up for bus tours, walking their dogs, eating ice cream cones, and snapping cell phone "selfies." Through the crowd, I spotted one security guard waving me over and yelling, "Hurry! He's in the cafeteria."

"Copy that," I said, throwing open the back ambulance doors and loading up the gurney with all the equipment I'd need to run a cardiac arrest—heart monitor; airway bag; the first-in bag with IV supplies, medications, and intubation tubes; a portable suction device; and a backboard to help move the patient and provide a solid surface on which to perform CPR.

As I worked, two park rangers arrived. "Grab the gurney and

I'll meet you inside," I said, pulling off the cardiac monitor and airway bag and directing the security guard to lead me inside.

"We're right behind you," said Janet, a law-enforcement ranger.

The best way out is through, I thought, following the security guard inside. At Yellowstone, the phrase meant responding to calls on snowy trails, on the rocky banks of rushing rivers, beside bison at geyser basins, and, that afternoon, in the Old Faithful Lodge. I held the cardiac monitor and airway bag as the security guard and I wove through tourists, and he told me, "It's not looking good and his wife is standing right there." As we neared, I saw a group of bystanders and heard the electronic voice of the automated external defibrillator (AED) saying, "No shock advised. Continue CPR . . ." and then the crowd parted before me. There was Edward Herzog lying on the floor. Now he was my patient.

I knelt, setting the cardiac monitor and airway bag down. A bystander, a vacationing doctor, gave me a quick report: "We were doing CPR for a few minutes and stopped just as you walked in. We also applied the AED."

"Any shocks delivered?" I asked, placing my first two fingers on the carotid artery in Edward's neck.

"No, sir," said the doctor, adding that he'd also disconnected Edward's insulin pump, meaning he was diabetic, and checked his blood sugar, which was elevated at 390.

I discovered Edward had a strong and rapid pulse, but his skin signs looked awful.

"Sir, wake up!" I said loudly, tapping Edward's shoulder.

He didn't respond. He just lay motionless with his eyes closed and a web of saliva hanging from his half-open mouth, so I tried another painful stimulus by pinching his shoulder.

Still nothing.

"What do you have?" asked Janet, arriving with the gurney. "And what do you need?"

"He's got a pulse but is unresponsive," I announced. "Let's launch a medevac helicopter. I need an oropharyngeal airway."

Janet radioed dispatch to request the helicopter as Brandon, another park ranger, rifled through the airway bag for an OPA. I threw on a stethoscope and continued checking Edward's ABCs. He had clear lung sounds but his breathing was rapid and shallow. What few sips of air Edward was inhaling certainly weren't reaching his lungs, and the nasal cannula that the security guard had placed to deliver 4 liters per minute of supplemental oxygen into his nose probably wasn't helping, either.

"I also need a bag-valve mask connected to high-flow oxygen," I said to Brandon.

Moving on to circulation, I found Edward's pulse continued to be strong and rapid; his skin signs were cool, dry, and pale; and his pupils were equal and reactive, which told me narcotics hadn't caused his collapse.

"Medevac has launched from West Yellowstone," Janet said, grabbing the backboard. "ETA twenty minutes to Old Faithful clinic."

As Brandon handed me the OPA and bag-valve mask, I instructed him and another ranger to apply a pulse oximeter to Edward's finger to check the oxygen saturation in his blood, and patch him up to the cardiac monitor to look at his ECG rhythm. As they immediately went to work, I tried to insert the OPA but Edward started to gag. I quickly removed it so he wouldn't vomit, and began ventilating him with the bag-valve mask. His chest rose and fell with each squeeze and I obtained a medical history from his wife, Annie, standing nearby.

"He has a history of high blood pressure, diabetes, elevated cholesterol, and coronary artery disease," she said, before adding that he'd also had stents inserted to keep the vessels supplying blood to his heart open and was on a laundry list of medications.

"Did he hit anything as he fell?" I asked, to determine if we needed to put Edward in full spinal immobilization.

"No," his wife said. "He had a large backpack on and he landed on it."

Edward didn't present with an abnormal ECG that I could treat; his pupils didn't suggest an overdose; his blood sugar was elevated but not likely the cause for him going unresponsive; and he had a strong radial pulse so it was unlikely that he was severely dehydrated. Thus I decided to transport him rapidly a half mile to the Old Faithful clinic, treating what I determined was his main, life-threatening problem—shortness of breath—with the bag-valve mask and high-flow oxygen.

"We'll stabilize him at the clinic and then transfer care to the flight team," I announced to everyone working with me.

When I finished speaking, the rangers burst into action, rolling Edward onto the backboard and applying safety straps. As they did, I continued delivering one breath every five seconds with the bag-valve mask and told his wife, Annie, that a ranger would drive her to the clinic. Moments later, we loaded Edward onto the gurney, wheeled him into the back of the ambulance, and took off with lights and sirens.

As we sped past spouting geysers and majestic pine forests, it dawned on me just how far—literally—I'd come since paramedic school.

After graduation, my fellow students from Class 36 scattered around the United States, most of them pursuing jobs with fire departments. We may have left the cozy classroom at the Walter S. Graf Center, but we still found ourselves taking more tests; this time, written firefighter exams in sprawling auditoriums and convention centers with thousands of other candidates as we came face-to-face with the lottery-like odds of getting hired.

While the competition was fierce and the hiring process inscru-
table at times, my classmates with both firefighter training and
paramedic licenses were all hired by fire departments in California
such as Culver City, Oxnard, Manhattan Beach, Garden Grove,
Bakersfield, and Escondido, and a few were picked up by fire departments in Washington, DC, and Texas. Other students worked for
private ambulance companies in Las Vegas, Santa Barbara, Compton, and Reno, among others.

Following school, I'd worked as a paramedic for a private ambulance company and had also had the honor of working as a skills
instructor in UCLA's EMT program (where, yes, I occasionally
failed students for not saying "BSI . . . scene safe"). I was then hired
by the National Park Service as a summer paramedic in the iconic
district of Old Faithful. There, my two great passions—the outdoors
and medicine—combined perfectly under the green and gray uniform, flat hat, and arrow-shaped badge. I was also able to attend
the National Park Service's Structural Fire Academy, where I learned
to fight fire, extricate patients from mangled vehicles, and perform
search and rescue missions in dark, smoked-filled rooms. At the
time of writing, I've also been hired to spend the winter working in
Yosemite as a firefighter/paramedic and am eagerly looking forward
to my start date.

Of course, working as a paramedic in a national park was vastly
different from the situation in Los Angeles, where, as Mr. Wheeler
once said, "You can't swing a dead cat without hitting a hospital."
In Yellowstone, our shortest transport time in the ambulance took
an hour and a half each way and routed us through three states.
We'd pick up our patients at Old Faithful (in Wyoming), transport
them out of the park via the West Yellowstone entrance (in Mon-
tana), then transfer them to another ambulance, staffed by paramedics, who'd transport the patients an additional hour to the
closest hospital (in Idaho). Using a "rendezvous" with a local fire

department in Idaho "shortened" our transport times and allowed us to return to Yellowstone to maintain 911 coverage.

While Yellowstone didn't have the high call volume Los Angeles did, most days working in a wilderness setting with extended transport times—an EMS system aptly described as "frontier medicine"—afforded me the chance to use a wider scope of practice, to enjoy a longer continuity of care with my patients, and to continue to grow my wings as a paramedic. The 911 calls themselves in Yellowstone were vastly different than in L.A., and we routinely used helicopters to transport critical patients out of the park. In Los Angeles, I treated patients who'd been shot, stabbed, or assaulted or who'd overdosed; in Yellowstone, I responded to calls for missing persons, patients suffering from heat exhaustion, strokelike symptoms, broken ankles, chest pain, allergic reactions, thermal burns, and vehicles that had rolled down forested hills. And there were also the cardiac and respiratory emergencies, such as Edward's collapse that afternoon.

As we raced to the clinic, I continued ventilating him with a bag-valve mask and we checked his blood sugar, which, as before, was elevated at 390. The oxygen and assisted ventilations helped and Edward became more responsive, moving all his extremities—which helped me rule out the possibility of a stroke—and, when he began blinking his eyes, I reassessed his mental status.

"Can you hear me, Mr. Herzog?" I said loudly. "Can you tell me where you are right now?"

Edward moaned weakly.

"You're in an ambulance at Yellowstone National Park," I said, comforting him. "You collapsed so we're taking you to the clinic and your wife will meet us there."

As Edward's respirations improved, I stopped using the bag-valve mask and switched him to a non-rebreather oxygen mask.

"Can you tell me your name?" I asked, continuing to assess his mental status.

"Edward . . ." he managed, "Herzog."

"Good!" I said, rechecking his vital signs and making sure his ECG rhythm hadn't changed. "Do you have any pain?"

"My chest," he said weakly. "And I'm cold."

As we pulled into the ambulance bay at the Old Faithful clinic, I quickly grabbed him a blanket.

The clinic was staffed by a physician assistant and two nurses, all of whom were waiting in the ambulance bay when we arrived. I quickly gave them a report and we moved Edward to a bed, started an IV, gave him aspirin to slow the ability of his blood to clot in the narrowed artery, administered morphine for the pain, and obtained a 12-lead ECG and another set of vital signs. The 12-lead ECG didn't show any acute ST elevation suggestive of a heart attack but Edward still needed rapid transport to a hospital to have his cardiac enzymes checked and to find the reason behind his collapse.

Presently, I heard the rhythmic *whoosh-whoosh-whoosh* of the helicopter arriving outside and Janet peeked her head into the treatment room to say, "The air ambulance is here."

I found Edward's wife, Annie, in the waiting room, filling out insurance information for her husband, and gave her a quick update on his condition and explained the reason we were flying him out in a helicopter.

When she asked if she could go with him, I explained that the weight limit on the helicopter wouldn't allow it. "But you can go see him now."

"Oh, good," she said, her eyes welling with tears.

"Mr. Herzog," I said, tapping his shoulder moments later, "I have someone very special here to see you!"

As Annie smiled and reached for her husband's hand, I was reminded that—as Captain Turner said—a paramedic's job is really about talking to people. Along with revealing a whole new side of our health care system, teaching me to save lives, and giving me a better appreciation for the country I call home, my experience working in EMS over the years has taught me that the best treatment is often making a personal connection with your patient. Thanks to EMS, my worldview has expanded and I've discovered that, beyond all our differences, people are all fundamentally the same. Like the Declaration of Independence states, we all have the right to life, liberty, and the pursuit of happiness and, as a paramedic, my job is to assist with that ever-important foundational element—good health.

Moments later, a flight nurse and paramedic walked in, wearing blue jumpsuits and white helmets. The physician assistant and I quickly informed them of Edward's chief complaint and of our interventions, then we handed them our paperwork and transferred him to their gurney.

"I'll see you at the hospital," Annie said to her husband, kissing him on the forehead and giving his hand a last good-bye squeeze.

Janet had arranged for one of the park volunteers to give Annie a courtesy ride to the hospital. "The Park Service always takes care of our guests," she said. "We never abandon anyone in an emergency."

I helped load Edward into the helicopter and gave him a friendly pat on the shoulder. "The flight crew will take good care of you," I said. "And be sure to come back to Yellowstone when you're feeling better."

"Never thought I'd be taking a scenic helicopter tour of the park," Edward joked in a barely audible voice and then thanked me for our care.

After Edward Herzog was moved into the helicopter, I donned a fluorescent vest and took my place at the entrance to an access road adjacent to the ranger station, to ensure that no one approached the area as the helicopter was taking flight. As the engines roared and rotors whooshed, tourists gathered to watch the helicopter lift off the ground. Among the spectators, I noticed a young boy. He stood next to his parents and their RV and was watching the helicopter take flight with the same spark of imagination and excitement on his face that I'd once had as a youth when I gazed at fire engines speeding by. Standing there, I couldn't help but smile and wonder what this boy's contribution to America would be one day. Perhaps he would become a park ranger. Or maybe he'd serve as a paramedic, firefighter, or police officer or join the military.

Watching him, I had an impulse to run over and tell him everything I'd discovered at paramedic school—about getting it done and that the best way out is through—but, as I saw him wave to the departing helicopter, leaping up and down with excitement, I knew he'd learn soon enough.

The important thing was that he was on his way.

Author's Note

In keeping with the Health Insurance Portability and Accountability Act (HIPAA) of 1996, identifying details of patients have been changed to protect their privacy. However, the chief complaint of the patients, the nature of the 911 calls, and the treatments I provided have not been changed. In addition, while the experience with my classmates, skills instructors, hospital staff, and Los Angeles Fire Department personnel was extremely positive, out of respect for their privacy, I have changed their names and some identifying details and, in some cases, have created composites of their combined personalities. I did not change the names of my primary instructors at UCLA, since they are well-known public figures and I thought it important to try to honor their work and legacy.

I used my class notes, daily journal entries, and internship evaluations to write this memoir. My hope is that it will provide readers with a sense of the rigorous training that paramedic students endure and will increase awareness and appreciation for this important profession. If this memoir kindles your interest in emergency medicine, and I hope it will, I encourage you to enroll in a CPR, first aid, or EMT class. Your life—to say nothing of the lives of others—will only benefit.

Acknowledgments

This memoir would not have been possible without the help of many colleagues, teachers, classmates, paramedics, firefighters, friends, and family members.

I am deeply indebted to my literary agent, Jane Dystel, and her business partner, Miriam Goderich, who helped bring the book proposal into the marketplace, navigate its sale, and then cheered me on at each and every stage of the writing and publishing process, offering valuable wisdom and support. Thank you!

I am grateful that this memoir found a home at Berkley Books and feel honored to be included among its impressive roster of authors and books. For her enthusiasm and belief in this project, I thank my hardworking editor, Shannon Jamieson Vazquez. Shannon brought a paramedic's precision to editing the manuscript—offering great ideas on how to inject air into the oxygen-deficient areas, how to splint hairline fractures of structure, and, overall, how to strengthen the book's pulse. Thanks also goes to Berkley's publisher, Leslie Gelbman; vice president and editorial director, Susan Allison; and to Sheila Moody for her copyediting work and Edwin Tse for his eye-catching cover design.

For their inspired instruction, mentorship, and passion for emergency medicine, I thank the staff at UCLA's Center for Pre-hospital Care with whom I've worked over the years: Dr. Baxter

Larmon, Todd LeGassick, Heather Davis, Brian Wheeler (and his golden retriever, Ophelia, whose wagging tail always eased the anxiety of test days), Nanci Medina, Justin McCullough, Michael Gudger, Dr. Atilla Uner, Lindsey Simpson, Barry Jensen, Jeff Pollakoff, Rosa Calva, Joseph Kalilikani, Quinn Bowyer, Case Kentis, Mark Malonzo, Ben Esparza, Michelle Torres, Davina Rios, and Anthony Mendoza.

For their friendship and for always pushing me to be my best, I thank all the members of Class 36. Facing a daily barrage of exams and skills tests, we held on to the one certainty—support from one another—to get it done and graduate. The constraints of a memoir dictated that I only include a few personalities but each of you inspired me daily, contributed equally, and the days we spent together will always be among my happiest.

My immense gratitude also goes to the Los Angeles Fire Department, which generously opened up the doors to Station 38 and hosted me as a paramedic intern. It was a privilege to serve alongside LAFD's professional cadre of paramedics and firefighters and my time there will be remembered fondly.

I owe particular recognition to my cousin Jamie Morse, an ER physician who clarified some of the procedures I witnessed during my clinical rotations, and to my uncle Griffin Morse, who provided the Spanish translations for two scenes. Thanks also goes to Renee Hetrick and Nanci Medina for their photography that appears in the book. I also wish to express my sincere appreciation to Dr. Richard Carmona, Peter Canning, Dr. Judy Melinek, T. J. Mitchell, and Dr. Paul Ruggieri who read an advance copy of the manuscript and provided promotional quotes.

Most important, I thank my family for their unbounded encouragement and love: the extended Grange and Morse clans and my immediate family—Mom, Dad, Kristine and Ola Johansson, Sean and Corie Grange, my niece, Lauren, and my nephews Bjorn, Finn, Hunter, and Taylor. Deflated after long days of writing, it was always such a pleasure to have my family to meet up with, and be re-inspired during an outdoor adventure or tasty meal.

Lastly, I'd like to say that each morning I feel grateful to wake up in a country where the bronze bell of democracy rings daily; where National Parks are sprinkled across the land like green jewels and where anything is possible for an entrepreneur or an artist with a creative idea. Thanks to the men and women serving in the military and to those working as firefighters, police officers, EMTs, paramedics, and park rangers who, together, stand ever-ready and ever-willing to keep our families safe. God Bless America!